I0520829

Run For Your Life

by

William McCollough

Copyright – 3rd Edition

© 2012 by William McCollough
.

All rights reserved. No portion of this book may be reproduced, stored in a retrieval system, or transmitted in any form or by any means - electronic, mechanical, photocopy, recording, scanning, or other - except for brief quotations in critical reviews or articles, without the prior written permission of the author. The author retains sole copyright to all contributions to this book.

Cover artwork titled "Running Athlete Silhouette Drawing Watercolor/Paint" is used by permission under non-exclusive, worldwide license granted by Adobe Corporation, 345 Park Avenue, San Jose, CA 95110-2704 for the cover of the book *Run For Your Life, A Journey of Mind, Body, and Spirit* by William McCollough.

"To give anything less than your best is to sacrifice the gift."

\- Steve Prefontaine

Contents

Foreword

by

Rachel Kopman

The focus I maintain with my clients as a Personal Trainer includes an innovative training style, concentrating on transforming not only the body but the mind as well. My training technique combines functional and traditional methods of working the body. In his book, *Run for Your Life,* Mr. McCollough applies the same sort of approach in that he gives us an in-depth view of transformation from a variety of viewpoints. Not only does he speak of the physical training aspects involved in gaining proper health and fitness goals, but he shares his story from the inner viewpoint. Although his nutritional advice for supporting a fitness goal, in this case reducing unwanted biomass, is rudimentary by design, he hits the high points and keeps the message simple. He provides a springboard from which the reader can launch a more detailed and personal study of what dietary considerations work best for them. He keeps the subject moving while providing an appropriate level intellectual stimulation for the reader.

Additionally, the reader gets to know exactly what the writer did in his journey from sedentary to active in conquering the demons of growing older. We all face an entropic universe where it is a fight just to maintain the health and fitness level we currently possess. In his simple approach to clearing the decks in his life, Mr. McCollough has laid down the proverbial breadcrumbs for others to follow. The reader is not required to guess what should be done; it is all right in front of you in plain English. He invites you along on his journey and encourages you to become bigger than your present self and make a positive change in your life.

Lastly, I need to acknowledge the inclusion of the mind – body relevance of this writing. As a Professional Trainer I know that what the mind can endure, the body can easily follow. My primary focus with beginning clients, and to a lesser degree my advanced clients, is to motivate them beyond their current level of desire to accomplish change. My biggest enemy is not the out-of-shape client but the mentally/emotionally weak client who will not internalize the experience I am imparting to them. The person who looks at training as just a physical endeavor, leaving the spiritual or energetic self behind is only getting half the benefit. If there is one thing I have learned, regardless of the type of client I have; whether they be a soft beginner or a hardened athlete seeking new levels of fitness, when the body and mind work together, the greatest results can be achieved.

I join Mr. McCollough in his invitation to make a change in yourself. I caution you, as he does, to always get professional help when taking on a new diet and exercise regimen. As with most changes in life, it will be uncomfortable at first, but I promise you the effort is well worth the benefits. Enjoy the reading and the "doing" on this wonderful excursion to better health.

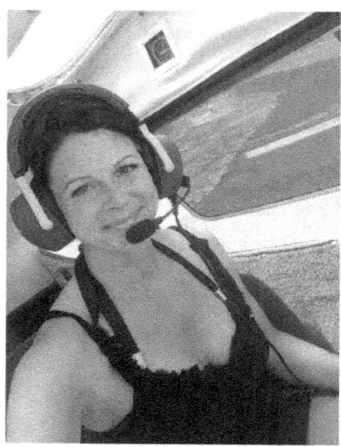

After a career in Law Enforcement, Rachel Kopman has been a Professional Personal Trainer for 6 years in Vancouver, Washington. Certified as a Theta practitioner, Ms. Kopman has expanded her resume to include Life and Personal Coach, and Healer helping people make meaningful changes in their lives. Pictured above, she also enjoys the life of an accomplished aviator. For more about Rachel, visit her at www.racchelann.com

Acknowledgements

The writing and publishing of any work is, of course, an arduous journey supported at various times by the people in our lives that matter. This being my first publication there are many people whom I want to acknowledge, however, time, and space on the page, will allow me to mention only the top of my list of folks to whom I am indebted.

I will start with my parents, William, and Harriet, who taught me perseverance, and to set my goals high. They told me many times that, "If you don't ask, you already have your answer," which I translated as meaning, "If you don't go for it, you won't get it."

Next, I would like to thank my two sisters, Joyce, and Barbara, for their undying support in all that I have done in my life. In my formative years they blazed a trail for me to follow and each imparted teachings necessary for me to stand in good stead while leading with my heart. Most of what I am in my adult life comes from them.

I must thank my daughters who have given me the greatest gifts in my lifetime. To my eldest kid, Cailin, I say thank you for getting me started on my running adventure and inspiring me to take on something extraordinary. And to my baby girl, Colleen, I send thanks for her help in exploring the spiritual side of this adventure and the art of "flowing."

Lastly, and certainly not least, I must acknowledge my good friend, coach, and mentor, Cindy Uskoski, for her love and hard work in getting me to act on my desire to write. Without her guidance, wisdom, and persistent encouragement, this book would not be in your hands right now.

Introduction

The purpose of this book is to shed some light on a journey from sedentary to active, and from lesser to greater on the way to increasing longevity and life enjoyment. This writing is aimed at two groups of folks. The first group is comprised of former athletes who have converted into the modern "couch potato" and are now unable to walk around the block or mow the lawn without gasping for breath. These people are usually the ones who still think they have "it," but do not anymore. The only way most guys in this group can tell if they have shiny shoes is to take the word of the shoeshine boy. The second group of folks I am talking to is comprised of younger people who do not want to end up that way.

I also want to attack some "truths" that we all have come to believe. By that I mean that there exists information that is documented by medical science and that is certainly factual in nature but is not "true" under all circumstances.

First, the information herein is mostly anecdotal in that a great deal of it is derived directly from my experience in conquering the monsters of aging and an increasingly sedentary lifestyle. Any information that I cannot directly vouch for in my story is documented and offered as a departure point for you to research for yourself and apply to your particular situation. I am not a doctor, trainer, exercise physiologist, or health expert of any kind.

However, I do claim that what you are about to read here is a method of turning the corner and heading in the direction of better health and enjoying a fuller life. Like anything you may read, it is certainly not "the" way of making a positive change physically, mentally, and spiritually in your life, but it is "a" way to do so. I have tried to make this writing informative without being too authoritative. I merely want to get your juices flowing and hopefully you will start thinking that a more active lifestyle is for you.

As background on me, you might be interested in knowing from where I am coming. I had been active for most of my life before descending into the abyss of poorer health. I played several varsity sports in high school and was fortunate enough to play football on the collegiate level in a Division 1 program.

After college I served in the United States Marine Corps for 21 years, so I kept in decent shape until I entered the private sector and had to "work" for a living. In 2001 I started to balloon up to over 300 pounds from an average weight of 235 pounds in the previous thirty years. I was always a "big" guy, but it was a real drain on my health having to carry sixty-five or more extra pounds around with me all the time. Of course, my skeleton, especially my knees and ankles, took a pounding, but the real victim of that excess weight was my old "trip hammer," pumping blood through the massive hulk that I had become.

I had gotten so big, even my mother told me directly, "You're too fat!" I started looking more critically at myself in the mirror and not liking what reflected back. But is that not like life itself, the Universe reflects back to us what we put out there and we can only change the world we live in by changing ourselves, starting with our perceptions.

After my mother took her shot, I realized my perception of my physical self was a lie. For many years I was not conscious of my size even though I had to change my entire wardrobe about every eighteen months to two years; an expensive proposition in any case. Each new wardrobe I acquired would "accommodate and conceal" my size and preserve my appearance for a time until a new set of clothes was needed. My point here is that without becoming aware of what is "true" in our lives, we will never make a change. This is linked to desire as well. To make any change in our lives we not only have to be aware, but we are required to want to make the change.

So, you can stop reading now if you are not really interested in at least becoming conscious about your physical being and making a positive change. What I found was that the mind, body, and spirit are intertwined so that a change in one will influence the others. As I mentioned above, this is an account of a journey that started for me when I became aware of what was happening to me physically. I discovered that my spiritual self and my ego wanted to come along for the ride as well. If you are interested in how a journey like this may change your life, read on. If you are still with me, welcome aboard and let us get started.

Chapter 1: Housekeeping

Before starting any physical exercise regimen, I must advise you to get a thorough check-up from your doctor, physician, healthcare professional, or whatever you may call them, especially if you are looking in the rear-view mirror at your 40th birthday. My doctor told me to work on dropping some weight before starting any strenuous routine. As indicated in the introduction, I was "a bit heavy," which is an understatement. I was tipping the scale at about 305 - 310 pounds when I concluded that I needed to do something to prolong my life and increase the quality of it before it was too late. I was on the road to a heart attack, or a stroke, or diabetes due to my eating and living habits. At a minimum I was not going to have a quality of life in my "golden years" if I continued on this path for much longer.

I was constantly fatigued, had aches and pains in my joints (especially the knees), had persistent headaches, had developed acid reflux, had a terrible time getting to sleep and staying asleep in the evening, and a worse time waking in the morning. Work was a survival event in that I had no energy to get efficiently through my workday and the afternoons were a foggy existence until I could get home to overeat for the third time that day at dinner.

When I went for my check-up, the advice I received from my doctor was to modify my diet in a way that would help reduce my weight. I had heard that before but when he got specific and told me about the effects of the fat I was storing all over my body, and most importantly, the fat that was accumulating around my heart, it got my attention. He told me that reducing the fat surrounding and compressing my heart would be like clearing the clutter from the workspace so that the work of pumping blood could be done more efficiently. Additionally, by dropping weight first, my exercise routine would be easier and more effective in eliminating weight and fat once I started working out. As I said, I had heard these words from a doctor before, but this time I heard the message, and it made sense. "When the student is ready, the teacher will appear," right?

Now that the subject of diet has been thrown out there, let us take a look at how you might want to go about modifying your diet, again, under the direction of a healthcare professional. I had done enough research to understand what my doctor was saying as he directed the initial effort for me to regain my health. Please note that the diet followed by one person is not necessarily what will work for another, but within certain "norms" everyone reacts to foods in the same way.

I had a friend in college who was convinced that if he did not eat "breakfast" food in the morning, or "lunch" and "dinner" foods respectively at their "proper times" each day, his health would suffer, and his life would be screwed up. As a student of Biology, I told him that the body does not know breakfast, lunch, and dinner; it only knows proteins, fats, and carbohydrates. It has been learned that the balance of these three food types is what is important in relation to what we need to do to be healthy at any point in our lives.

You should know that proteins are the basic building blocks of life. Without protein in the diet, babies could not grow, or adults could not repair damaged cells. Without going into how proteins are formed and a discussion of amino acids and peptide bonds, etc., I will just say that proteins are needed to maintain a healthy state of being. Proteins, either animal or vegetable are similar when the body uses them. However, you may want to monitor how proteins are packaged. A 6-ounce steak will have plenty of protein along with nearly an equal amount of fat, whereas the same size piece of salmon gives you about the same protein with less than half the fat. It is not necessarily true that eating fat makes you fat, but you may want to keep an eye on what kinds of protein you are eating.

As long as you are getting an adequate amount of protein in your diet, I believe that carbohydrates and fats are more important to look at from the viewpoint of weight control. A careful study of what your body needs is essential to make the proper adjustments to positively affect your diet and health. Here is what worked for me.

I took a good look at my eating habits from a consumer's standpoint. The old saying, "What you eat, you are," is true, but for me what was more true was how I ate. I was eating three huge meals every day at about the same time each day without regard to how hungry I was. I do not think we humans were created to "consume mass quantities," to quote the Coneheads of Saturday Night Live fame. Most of us eat like it will be our last meal at every meal and we have a challenging time understanding why we are getting heavier or not reducing weight even when we exercise.

There is a simple formula for regulating your body weight if you are interested in weight loss. Our bodies know this simple rule, but we do not. If the number of calories coming in (due to eating) exceeds the number going out (due to exercise), we gain weight. If the number of calories going out exceeds the number coming in, we lose weight. So, if you do not exercise and want to lose weight, here is the secret; "Eat less."

That is not always easy; in fact, it is never easy to eat less when we have conditioned ourselves to consume at any certain level of food intake. What I learned to do was to slow down during mealtime and allow my body to signal my brain that I had indeed consumed enough to turn off the "hungry light" inside me. When I did that, I ate less. Now, I am not a diet Guru, nor am I inclined to explain the psychology behind why we do things that are detrimental to our health, like overeating, I simply know that when I slowed down at mealtime, I ate less food.

I also learned to eat when I was hungry. This led me to eat smaller meals more times a day to meet the energy demand at any particular time. Generally speaking, I now eat five to six meals a day on average: three "main" meals and a snack meal between them. This tends to keep my blood sugar at a more constant level throughout the day and I enjoy having the energy necessary to finish strong in the afternoons.

After I was able to appreciate the art of listening to my body a bit more, I decided to target certain things in my diet that repressed my ability to lose weight. If you go this route, you will have to have some discipline, but it will pay off. I stopped consuming sugars, breads, dairy products, alcohol, and caffeine (I will break this down further in a minute). The foods and beverages represented by the list above had become a comfort to me. Psychologically, I "felt" better when I ate this stuff, although my physical body was telling me otherwise. It was no problem for me to overindulge on any of these substances. I could easily drink a six-pack of beer every night when I got home from work in the evening (before, during and after my evening meal) – or a large part of a case on the weekends – all by myself.

I was so bad, I remember years ago, I asked my spouse at the time, "Did you have a party that I don't know about?" as I observed the number of beer bottles in the recycle bin in the garage. "Who drank all that beer?" I asked her.

"You did!" she said as she walked away laughing.

For years I was completely unconscious of my beer intake. I would also routinely eat an entire package of "store-bought" cookies or a half gallon of ice cream in a single sitting. Can you see me sitting there, wolfing down a carton of Rocky Road while watching the evening news? Ah, the good old days.

In fact, I was slowly killing myself with all that "comfort food" I was consuming. Considering the physiology of the subject, can you imagine what that type of intake was doing to my liver – or my pancreas? "Over the lips and passed the gums, look-out body, here it comes." Anything that we overeat takes a toll on the liver, especially those foods I was overeating, because the liver ends up chemically processing everything we ingest. Let us take a look at what these culprits are up to as they enter our bodies.

Sugars: The term "sugar" refers to a class of edible crystalline carbohydrates; mainly sucrose, lactose, and fructose, characterized by a sweet flavor. In processed foods, sugar almost exclusively refers to sucrose, which primarily comes from sugar cane and sugar beet. Other sugars are used in industrial food preparation, but are usually known by more specific names — glucose, fructose or fruit sugar, high fructose corn syrup, etc. [1]

Obviously, to eliminate this menace to the body I stopped eating all sugars in cookies, candies, soft drinks, etc., but I also gave up the natural sugars in fruits as well. There are no "good" or "bad" sugars; sugar is sugar. I have since allowed myself to go back to eating fresh fruits in moderation, but initially, I cut out all sugars including the sugars in fruits. Why did I do this? Well, sugars are simple carbohydrates, and the body will follow the path of least resistance and break down these carbohydrates first leaving the more complex carbohydrates for storage in the body.

I also learned that a major drawback of sugar ingestion is that it can rapidly raise the insulin level in the body. An influx of sugar into the bloodstream upsets the body's blood-sugar balance triggering the pancreas to release insulin, which the body uses to keep blood-sugar at a constant and safe level. Increased insulin promotes the storage of fat, so, when you eat foods high in sugar, you are setting yourself up for weight gain, specifically a fat gain, which is a major contributor to heart disease. Additionally, an increased insulin level inhibits the release of growth hormones which can depress the immune system. The last thing anyone needs is a depressed immune system.[2]

---

[1] http://www.freebase.com/view/en/sugar

[2] Larrow, A. (2010) Sugar's effect on your Health, from http://www.drlarrownd. com /node/128

Unfortunately, nearly all processed food on the market today has sugar in it. Avoiding sugar completely takes some effort. Initially I was satisfied to drop the sugar that I could in eliminating things I habitually ingested each day like soft drinks and desserts. But soon I started reading labels on everything I bought at the grocery store. Now, when I am "comparison shopping," I do not always buy the brand name or the cheapest item. The product with the least sugar added goes into my basket! I still had a craving for the "white powder" since my sweet tooth was well endowed, so for several weeks after going cold turkey, I was a little edgy, so to speak. I loved the sweetness, but I did not want to make the mistake of using the standard sugar substitutes (I will refrain from naming them, but you know the ones I am talking about) because they can have some other effects including the tendency to have your body hold onto unwanted weight.[3]

You see, I learned that not all carbohydrates are created equal; in fact, they behave quite differently in our bodies. The glycemic index (GI) describes this difference by ranking carbohydrates according to their effect on our blood glucose levels.[4] Choosing low GI carbohydrates, in other words the ones that produce small fluctuations in our blood glucose and insulin levels, is the secret to long-term health and the key to sustainable weight loss. And by reducing your weight you will reduce your risk of heart disease and diabetes as well.[5] Since my sweet tooth needed

---

[3] Manzella, D., Can Artificial Sweeteners Make You Gain . from http://diabetes. about.com/od/nutrition/qt/artificialsweet.htm

[4] http://web.mac.com/brand.it.now/ Halo_The_Good_Sweetener_1. /halo01. html

[5] ArticleBase, How to Lose Inches Off Your Waist –Three Steps to Help You Reduce The Amount of Sugar You Eat! From http://www.articlesbase.com/ nutrition-articles/how-to-lose-inches-off-your-waist-three-steps-to-help-you-reduce-the-amount-of-sugar-you- eat-4733068.html

to be satisfied, I did end up looking for a substitute sweetener that had a low GI and found Xylitol to be satisfactory for use in sweetening my drinks, such as tea (naturally decaffeinated, of course), or on my oatmeal, and for use in cooking. Xylotol helped me satisfy my sweet tooth while not ingesting high GI sugary foods.

Bread: Bread is one of the oldest prepared foods. For about 10,000 years, humans have been making breads along with planting vegetables in shifting from the "hunter – gatherer" existence to a more agrarian society. The result is more starch in the diet.[6]

Overeating carbohydrate foods can prevent a higher percentage of fats from being used for energy, and lead to a decrease in endurance and an increase in fat storage. Eating processed grains in bread can trigger the body to store fat. For millions of years before the agrarian age, the human diet consisted primarily of proteins and fats from eating animal flesh. When meat was scarce due to animal migration or a poor hunting season, humans ate what they could to survive which meant eating foods from the plant kingdom – comparatively high carbohydrate foods. Their bodies would take this change in food intake as a signal that times were lean, and more storage had to occur to survive.

Genetically speaking, our bodies are closely related to our ancient ancestors metabolically, and today our bodies respond in the same way in that additional carbohydrates in the diet will increase insulin and trigger the body to store fat. So, bread was out!

---

[6] http://en.wikipedia.org/wiki/Bread

Dairy: Milk has around fifteen grams of sugar per 8-ounce serving. Cheese will be higher in the amount of fat and protein per unit volume. Some yogurts have around fifty grams of sugar per 12-ounce serving. Most of the carbohydrates in dairy foods come from sugars. Dairy products are roughly 65% carbohydrates and 35% protein. Carbohydrates in dairy foods are mostly lactose.[7] My avoidance of sugar had to include dairy products because dairy products are high carbohydrate foods, which contribute to weight gain when ingested regularly. We have already discussed the effect carbohydrates have on weight and fat gain in the human body. Dairy was out!

Alcohol: Alcohol negatively impacts the blood-sugar level in the body and causes the increased production of insulin. Like sugars, alcohol can cause an increase in insulin levels that hurt the effort for weight loss. I was a beer drinker, so besides the alcohol, I was ingesting excess carbohydrates with every beer I drank. Enough said.

Caffeine: Many people have the popular misconception that caffeine will help them lose weight. Unfortunately, the opposite is true. Drinking caffeinated beverages or taking pills containing caffeine ultimately stimulates an increased appetite for sweets and fatty foods. Caffeine triggers a roller coaster ride of elevated blood sugar, due to ingesting additional sweets, and produce stress hormones that thwart our efforts to stick to the diet regimen.[8] Again, enough said.

Regardless of the physiological effects that these foods have on the body once ingested, they all had one other

---

[7] Dolson, L. Carbohydrate Counts of Dairy Products from http://lowcarbdiets. about.com/od/whattoeat/a/dairycarbs.htm

[8] Livermore, B. 1991. Caffeine Boosts Eating Disorders. Health. June: 16.

thing in common in making it difficult for me to lose weight; they had an addictive effect on me, and I was unconsciously over-ingesting them. I also learned that I was more likely to eat these things when I was watching television, a sedentary activity, and an activity which promoted less awareness of my eating habits. So, now I listen to music during mealtimes instead of watching TV.

One last habit I formed while fighting back on my eating habits was not eating after 7:00 PM. Drinking water was all right, but ingesting nothing solid after that time helped me be more conscious of what I was eating. It also set up a healthy hunger for breakfast the next morning. I was less likely to skip or skimp on eating breakfast which I feel is an important meal. I do not understand folks who do not eat breakfast. How do they get started in the morning?

Another little trick I would use during the day to curb unconscious eating was to brush my teeth after each meal. It kept me from eating foods or snacks that would "dirty" my teeth and it brightened my smile too. What it boils down to is becoming conscious of both good and bad habits. We cannot really break a "bad" habit; we must replace it with a "good" habit. I have found that if I can replace a bad habit with a good habit for three weeks (just 21 days), usually, that "good" habit will become my new habit. The point here is the more you are aware of what you are eating; the better able you are to eat the right things or to not eat things that are bad for you and your diet.

Finally, I have to say that this first step can be a doozy! Anytime you make changes in your habits, especially in your diet, your body will react to it. Initially, your body will tell you that you had better not do this and will present all sorts of strange feelings, aches and pains, and just plain internal havoc to get you to go back to your old eating habits. You will swear that you are getting sick, or you are having a heart attack, your lungs are going to collapse, you have a brain tumor causing a headache that you never felt before, or something life shattering will happen if you don't go back on your "normal" diet. In essence, your body is a spoiled brat that wants things its own way. After starting my new diet, I had several episodes with my breathing when I reclined; I was nauseous; I had a short bout with diarrhea; and a caffeine withdrawal headache for about a week after I started eating differently. My body tried everything in the book to convince me that I needed that sugar, alcohol, caffeine, etc.

As I did on occasion, you will give into your "brat" body and sneak something or other that you are trying to eliminate. You may feel guilty that you could not stick it out, but you will feel "better" after that sugar fix or whatever you had to have. Do not beat yourself up and revert to going unconscious in monitoring your diet, just start anew and get back to work. Nothing h. is absolute, just get back on track and keep going. Little slip ups will not matter in the long run (pun intended). But that is the acid test that should tell you that you are on the right path with the modified diet. If your sugar craving stops when you sneak that treat that you normally ate or your headache subsides when you down that cup of coffee, you will know that the cause of the ailment was simply the change in diet. Stick with it and ride out the withdrawal period. You will be glad you did.

Once I got over the hump and my consistency with the diet solidified, I realized a significant weight loss of about ten pounds a month for the first four months. Even though I still had a way to go before my ideal weight was realized, I felt much lighter (indeed, I was much lighter) and was ready to start exercising. As a side note, I lost over sixty pounds in a little over four months primarily due to my change of diet.

Just about the time I was starting to monitor what I was eating, my oldest daughter called me and asked if I would like to train and run with her in her first half marathon. Perfect timing: I accepted.

Now that my diet was coming under control, it was time for me to think about the transition from sedentary to active. I knew I needed to do some running to prepare for participation with my darling daughter in the half marathon, but I really was not properly equipped. I figured all I needed was a pair of shoes and a road to run on and I would be set. Is there any more to it than that?

Chapter 2: Gearing Up and Getting Started

I mentioned in the last chapter that all one needs to start shaping up via the use of long-distance running was a pair of shoes and a road to run on. Let me set the table a bit better. You are nearly ready to start, in my opinion, when you have had your medical check-up, taken control of your diet, got your weight change started in a downward mode, and committed to a consistent training regimen. There are also some safety considerations that will be covered in the next chapter, and I want to cover some of the "truths" surrounding aging and exercise. But for now, let us look simply at the physical requirements of this undertaking.

One of the last steps in this preparation process is outfitting yourself for the road ahead. The foundation of the gear necessary for this trip is obviously your shoes. The importance of getting the right shoe for you is emphasized by the fact that research done on runners tells us that a load equaling 1.5 to 5 times our body weight (on average) is absorbed by our legs on each stride we take while running. This is compounded in the feet to a reported 6 to 10 times body weight on each foot-strike. This repetitive loading will cause damage if not accommodated by having the right shoe on to help absorb that impact and minimize the cumulative trauma to the body.[9]

---

[9] Katherine O'Leary, MPT; Kristin Anderson Vorpahl, MPT, OTR; Bryan Heiderscheit, PT, PhD; "Effect of Cushioned Insoles on Impact Forces During Running" from http://www.engr.wisc.edu/ groups/nmbl/ pubs/ japma08 _oleary.pdf

As you may know, not all athletic shoes are the same. Some are designed for walking, some for cross training, some for running, etc. Although I believed that I was able to run in any type of athletic shoe, because, for years, that is what I did, it is best to make an investment in your feet, knees and hips by buying a shoe that is designed for what you want to do. I know what you are thinking, *"There goes a wad of cash for a fancy pair of shoes,"* but you do not necessarily have to purchase the high-end running shoe to get a great shoe and one that fits you and your needs. A decent shoe may cost $80 to $120 at most sporting goods stores. You might be surprised to know that specialty running stores are not always the most expensive place to get your gear and they usually offer some sort of expertise beyond the average sales-person pitch.[10]

Let me give you some guidelines on shoe selection and why you need to talk with someone who knows what they are talking about when it comes to running. Now remember, I told you I am not an exercise physiologist, or trainer of any type. Some of what I am telling you is just the information I considered while selecting my treads. We all have a unique body and special needs, but, again, within certain norms most humans fall into general categories. If you have podiatric anomalies, then you should consult a specialist on what to put on your feet. A "specialist" is not necessarily a physician (like a podiatrist) but can be an exercise physiologist, biomechanist, or specialized trainer. They may know better what is going on with your feet, among other body parts, and how you use them while you are running, than your doctor. Be areful either way in whichever person's advice you follow.

---

[10] **How to choose running shoes, from http://www.rei.com/expertadvice/ articles/running+shoes.html**

I happened to be able to consult with the owner of VA Runners in Woodbridge, Virginia, Jeff Van Horn.[11] Jeff was at that time Northern Virginia's foremost authority and expert on running biomechanics, running injuries, and running shoes. He holds a B.A.A. degree in Sports Medicine and Exercise Science. When I first met him, I did not know who I was talking to, but within ten seconds I realized this guy would set me straight. Jeff took the time to educate me on various considerations involved in getting into the right shoe. Oddly enough, price was not a consideration either way, up or down. His mission was to get me fitted in the shoe that was right for me. Part of the education process was to have me understand that we all fall into one of three categories of body type: ectomorph, mesomorph, or endomorph.

Very quickly, an ectomorph is a typical skinny person having a light build with flexible joints and lean muscles. Usually, ectomorphs have long thin limbs with stringy muscles and shoulders tending to be thin and narrow in width. Running is usually a more natural exercise for them. A mesomorph has a large bone structure, large muscles, and a naturally athletic physique. Mesomorphs are the best body type for athletic training and find it quite easy to gain and lose weight. They are naturally strong, having the perfect platform for building muscle. This group of folks can easily adapt to a running regimen to complement their training routine. The endomorphic body type is solid but generally soft. Endomorphs gain fat very easily and are usually of a shorter build with thick arms and legs. Their muscles are strong, especially in the upper legs. Endomorphs find they are naturally strong in leg exercises like squats but must work a little harder to

---

[11] VA Runner http://www.varunner.com/?page_id=19

get into a running regimen.[12] So, which body type are you? Given the information above you should easily be able to identify your body type. You may be a combination of these types, and you should optimize your diet and training to suit whichever type you are. The point I want to make here is that no matter what your body type is, you can create the healthy and attractive physique that you desire.

In addition to knowing your body type, you must understand that each type presents a different equation when it comes to running. The main consideration is your joint structure. We humans have either a stable or an unstable gait in our running motion due to how our joints are constructed. Stable joints are less flexible and tend to hold alignment better under stress or during exercise. Unstable joints are looser and more flexible, and less able to hold alignment when stressed. As you might imagine, ectomorphs have a less stable joint structure while mesomorphs and endomorphs tend to have more stable joints.

The science of constructing an athletic shoe to support these types of joint structures is what the big shoe manufacturers invest a lot of time and money into. The different manufacturers all do an excellent job in making shoes that are beneficial to the average runner out there. What manufacturer is the best? I could not say, because different strategies of shoe building work for different people. And that is the point here. Regardless of which brand name you like or how much money you can spend, you just will not know which shoe is for you until you

---

[12] **Body type: ecto- meso- endomorph article, from http://www.muscleand strength.com/articles/body-types-ectomorph-mesomorph-endomorph.htm**

investigate thoroughly and get the right advice for your particular body type and running style. Here is what Jeff did for me.

When I met Jeff, we started out talking about nutrition and energy to sustain me on the run. I needed to get some information on what nutritional supplements would work to keep me going during the training runs and during the half-marathon itself. I will share the nutrition information in a later chapter. Our conversation shifted to shoe performance and Jeff quickly discerned that I might need a review of what I was putting on my feet before running. I will not get into brand names here as that would be a disservice to you, the manufacturers, and to the integrity of this writing.

As I said previously, each of us must make our own decision about the gear we get. Simply put, Jeff educated me on the fact that within certain norms we are all running in a unique way. Like anything in life, when it comes to running, there are different strokes for different folks. Some of us are more stable and neutral, while others have quirks in their gaits to be tweaked or corrected by employing different support structures that exist in different shoes. My guess is that since I was a former athlete, I presented less of a challenge to Jeff's diagnostic skills.

After measuring my feet for proper size, he put me in a pair of light weight "test" shoes and had me jog on the sidewalk in front of the store. This first pair of shoes was designed for this test alone as they were very flexible and would help to reveal the characteristics of my foot-strike, knee alignment, etc. I ran straight away from him and straight at him as he observed my gait. Jeff told me I was a neutral, stable runner in his estimation, and he took me back inside to select several different shoes that would serve my needs. He had me try each of them on, instructing me to be sure that I tapped my heel to "snug" my foot to the rear of the shoe before tying the laces. This allows the shoe to mount properly to the foot and takes unnecessary pressure off the toes. He also checked the room for my toes and explained that the metatarsal bones near the ball of the foot need room to spread out while being supported to properly absorb the shock of the foot-strike on each stride (remember those impact numbers I shared earlier).[13] [14]

The ball of the foot and pain in that area is something we will cover in a later chapter. For now, I will just mention that ill-fitting shoes most certainly contribute to trouble and injury while running any distance. Again, I ran with each suggested pair of shoes while Jeff observed to see if anything had changed. I was able to feel each shoe for fit and comfort while running. I came to a decision easily when presented with a quality selection of shoes.

I think I have made my point. Get some decent shoes before you tear your feet and knees apart. Remember when you were a kid, and you got a new pair of shoes? They fit exactly right, and they made you feel like you could run far and fast if you wanted to. I got a pair of PF Flyers when I was ten years old, and I swear I could run faster and jump high enough to clear the back fence. That was almost all psych then, but the point is you do not

---

[13] Foot - metatarsal information, from http://ezinearticles.com/?Metatarsal-Running-Pain&id=1003721

[14] Metatarsal Stress information, from http://www.runnersrescue.com/ Metatarsal_Stress_Fracture_Running.htm

want to have to push through a run with shoes that do not at least feel good to be running in.

Remember, let the shoes do the work. Do not modify your gait or how your foot strikes the ground to compensate for any discomfort you may be feeling. If you have a need for support somewhere in your shoe to properly align your ankle or knee, your chosen expert, like Jeff, will know how to correct it and advise you accordingly. If you have pronation (inward roll of the ankle) or supination (outward roll of the ankle), the misalignment of your ankle may not allow for strong enough support while running. Damage to your ankle may occur over time or you may suffer an acute ankle injury (a sprain or total ligamental rupture) during a run. These types of injuries are best treated or prevented using orthotic inserts.[15]

Be aware that an incorrect alignment of your ankle could affect your knees and hips as well. The misalignment will translate up through the structure of the leg and depending on your particular joint configuration, you could feel discomfort in either the knee, or hip, or both. Sometimes all it takes is a simple adjustment in the shoe to clear up some serious discomfort. In any event, do not adjust your gait to the shoe; adjust the shoe to your gait.

Now we will shift to the upper body. Posture is important, even in running – and maybe especially so. Many people will run with poor posture which tends to increase stress in the body. Running upright, with your head up and shoulders back is preferable to being tight in the shoulders

---

[15] Pronation / Supination Information, from http://www.runnersworld.com /article/0,7120,s6-240-319-327-7727-0,00.html

and bent into the run. Relaxing the shoulders will help dissipate tension and allow the arms to swing freely and fluidly on each stride.

Keeping the head up and shoulders back also promotes breathing by aligning the neck and trunk so that the airway stays optimally open. We will discuss breath control later, but suffice to say, we all breathe easier when our posture is correct. Try taking a few breaths with your shoulders hunched forward and your head bent downward. Feel the tension in your chest cavity and how your lungs are restricted. Continue breathing and straighten up so that your shoulders are back, your chest is relaxed, and your head is upright. Feel the difference? If correct posture makes it easier for you to breathe while you are sitting there reading this, imagine how critical it is when you are running, and every breath needs to be at its fullest for you to sustain that activity. "Straighten up and fly right."

Arm swing is important too. The tendency is to hold tension in your arms as you run. If you are running with clenched fists, you are increasing the tension in your arms. This translates to the entire body via the shoulders, torso and mid-section which makes running much more difficult. Let your arms swing in a relaxed motion and if you find yourself starting to clench your fists, relax your arms by your sides and shake them out. Keep your fingers loose by lightly touching your fingertips to your thumb tips. This technique helps me in preventing the tension from building.

We have only scratched the surface of the body mechanics arena here so you may want to do some more research to better understand your particular body alignment questions. I have provided all my sources in the references in this publication to give you some points to depart from. Just remember one thing, do not try to diagnose yourself. Even a minor problem can translate into real trouble if you do not know what you are doing. Even if you think you know what you are doing, I advise you to get the opinion of an outside observer who knows what he or she is talking about. A structurally sound house cannot be built on a weak or crooked foundation. Building a strong body falls under the same principle. If you want to make this a pleasurable experience, then make your foundation strong right from the beginning. This is supposed to be fun, and it will not be if you are in constant pain due to ill-fitting shoes or poor posture. With even a minor understanding of your body mechanics, you can avoid the pitfalls when starting this new workout regimen. Put your best foot forward, so to speak – pun intended.

There are some other pieces of gear that you may want to consider that will make your running workouts more manageable. They are not "necessary," but once you use them, you will never run without them.

Sunglasses: While pursuing outdoor activities most of us like to wear something to protect our eyes from the damaging or discomforting effect of nature. Sunglasses are designed to protect the eyes primarily from bright sunlight and other high-energy visible light. They also help cancel out the invisible and harmful UV rays from the sun. You also may consider getting a pair that wrap around your face to maximize the protection from sun and especially from dust blowing into your eyes from the sides. They need to fit close to your face, which may feel a bit uncomfortable at first, but not too close to block any type of air exchange. It tends to get foggy under your glasses if no air can circulate up under the lenses. A good pair of lightweight running shades can run you anywhere from $35 to $200 depending on what you want. Regardless of price, get a pair of glasses with polarized lenses for best protection. I got mine for $35 (plus tax, of course) at a health and fitness expo before one of the half marathons I ran, and they work great.

Runner's Pack: A runner's pack is a fanny pack that can carry some necessities on the run. Designed to stay close to the body to reduce flapping up and down, these packs are really great for carrying your identification, some nutrient packs, or even a cell phone while you run. Fitting tightly around the waist, these little packs are made to stretch to accommodate a fair number of goodies. Some are even designed with built-in water bottles for those long training runs. The price of these packs are as little as $9 ranging to $45 on Amazon, again, depending on what you want to take along.

Armband Carrier: I am sure you have seen folks out there listening to their tunes with an iPod tucked neatly into an elastic armband (I know iPods are passe', but I still have mine). These cost between $6 and $20 allowing you to carry your cell phone, a more useful choice than an iPod, if you do not want to use a runner's pack.

Hydration Packs: If you are up for carrying a little weight on your   training workouts, a hydration pack is great for providing either water or your favorite brand of sports-themed beverage product on the run. There are a variety of hydration systems depending on what is most comfortable for you. Some are worn like a backpack having a hose that can be clipped to the front strap so you can suck up the liquid you need with little effort. With many models to choose from, these packs range from $30 to $100 at most sporting goods stores and camping supply houses. Others are set up as a "butt pack" style belt with holsters for hydration flasks or bottles.

The minimalist hydration packs can be worn while running with little flapping. You can snug them down to stay with your body while in motion. These packs also have some storage pouches to put your ID, car keys, cell phone, etc. away while running. Still another type of hydration system accomplishes the task of carrying the liquid of choice by means of a handheld bottle. The bottle or flask slips into a small pouch with a strap that you slide your hand into so you can carry it without having to use a great amount of energy for gripping.

You may be wondering what is better for you during a long run, water, or sports drink? You will need to replenish yourself energy-wise during longer runs to sustain the pace you want. You have a choice of packing and using energy chews (sort of like super-powered gummy bears) or drinking a sports drink that will supply extra energy as well as hydration. If you are not supplementing your energy level with some sort of nutrient food (energy chews or the like), then I would suggest you find a drink that will give you some electrolyte and carbohydrate intake to put in your hydration pack. Again, there are several brands to choose from and just like finding the right shoe; everyone has a favorite product to use. Research and experiment with several different methods to find the one that works best for you.

Hats: "To wear or not to wear; that is the question." There are two schools of thought about wearing a hat while exercising. Arguments on both sides cite various factors. The belief that most of the heat escapes the body through your neck and head has been debunked. What is more reasonable is to say that you lose heat from your head in proportion to its surface area relative to your body size. I can tell you that on frigid days you will lose less heat through your head when wearing a hat. Conversely, on hot days a hat will tend to hold heat in the body that would have escaped from the head. There is the consideration that wearing a hat shields your noggin from direct sun which helps to protect you and keep you a bit cooler. On hotter days I soak my hat in water before a run to increase the amount of liquid for evaporation to promote cooling. I think it mainly boils down to personal comfort.[16]

Well, that is my cut at the gear list. You may find other things that serve you on the run while you adjust to your new activity. We will talk about some other things that will help you prepare for the event of your choosing. For now, you have a good idea of the gear that is available and what you may want. Next, we will talk about safety.

---

[16] Body Heat Loss information, from http://www.guardian.co.uk/science /2008/dec/17/medicalresearch-humanbehaviour

Chapter 3: Safety

In this short chapter we will discuss common practices for staying safe while pursuing the activity of long-distance running. Certain elements of this pursuit are critical when it comes to keeping safe. Factors such as the area in which you run, the time of day at which you run, or even the weather are things to be considered if you intend to manage the risks down to a reasonable level.

Distance: It is particularly important to allow your body to adjust to this activity. Starting out at shorter distances and working your way up to the desired distance, whether it is a 5K or a marathon, will help you achieve your goal safely and more quickly. There is such a thing as over training. We will cover that later. The idea is to take it easy at first, then let the clutch out and start rolling faster and farther as time goes on.

Location: Where you run is as important as how far you run. It is much more preferable to run in a place that is not adjacent to vehicular traffic. If a park or a community trail, or even a bike path along a road is available, I advise you to use it. These areas are away from cars and trucks whizzing by at break-neck speed. These facilities are also usually areas where the air is fresher and relatively pollution free. There is nothing worse than puffing hard to supply your body with the oxygen it needs when the air is laden with exhaust fumes from the daily traffic. Unless you run early, before the traffic is heavy, you will appreciate being away from internal combustion engines when you run.

Pick a nearby park or recreation area that will allow you to run unmolested by motorists. A bike trail or hiking trail may be suitable but check out the trail in advance to be sure that the road surface is fairly consistent and evenly graded. Roots and rocks tend to play havoc on unsuspecting toes and ankles. Many towns have bike paths along major thoroughfares allowing community use while walking, bike riding or running. If you live near a Rails-to-Trails Conservancy area where an old railroad bed is converted to a riding / hiking trail, you have an ideal opportunity to put on some mileage in a safe place. You can even run at the local high school track. It might be boring, but it is safe.

If you do not have these types of areas handy to your home, and you are forced to run along roads with traffic, use your head. Wear brightly colored clothing with reflective surfaces incorporated into them to improve a driver's visibility of you, especially in the wee hours of the morning or in the evening. Always run facing the oncoming traffic so that you can see how a vehicle is behaving while it approaches. Drivers do not pay enough attention to ensure that you will be seen, even when wearing proper clothing. A driver's inattention at the wrong time could be a recipe for disaster for a runner, so keep alert to what each car that passes you is doing. You can always jump out of the way at the last second if you see the car veering off the road toward you. I have had to do this more than once to keep from being mowed down by some knucklehead with a motor vehicle.

In deciding where to train, you might want to talk to other runners or visit a local sports store. They probably can point you to some accurately measured courses that are safe for your workouts.

Time of Day: If you must run at extreme ends of the day due to your schedule, or if you need to run in the early morning when the temperature is lower, then be smart and prepare yourself to accommodate low-light situations.

Obviously, visibility is especially important while running. Not only visibility of you to others, but also your ability to see your surroundings should be considered. It is suggested you wear some sort of light system including a head lamp (a specialized flashlight that attaches to your head by an elastic band) for seeing ahead of you and a rear blinker light (attached to some part of you) for visibility of you from the rear. Be familiar with the running course as well so that you will not be surprised by any unexpected obstacles in your path.

Weather: There is nothing wrong with running during inclement weather. Rain will not hurt you, just be careful of your footing while running in the rain. Running in extreme hot or cold weather can be detrimental to your health if you are not acclimatized. The former U.S. women's record holder for the Boston Marathon, Desiree Davila, did a great deal of her running in Tempe Arizona as a student at Arizona State University. Year-round outdoor training in Arizona presents a challenge for would-be runners as the temperature often rises above one hundred degrees Fahrenheit by 8:00 AM. Desiree had to adjust her day around times when the temperature was bearable for putting in mileage.

Wintry weather can be challenging as well. If you are not used to running in wintry weather, be careful about heading outside to run below freezing. The extreme cold can cause discomfort to your airways and lungs. You will not necessarily freeze them, but you will have to get used to the cold, dry air moving in and out of your airway. Care should be taken in extreme cold to protect exposed skin from freezing. To stay comfortable in frigid weather, wear a microfiber shirt as a first layer, followed by a breathable windbreaker, gloves or mittens, and a hat. Begin by running into the wind, not with it, which will keep you from sweating to much starting out. Sweat is bad in winter, as water robs heat from your body up to twenty-five times faster than trapped air does.

Communicate: One of the best things you can do for yourself is tell someone where you are going to run, explaining the route and how long you expect to be running. We can all learn from Aron Ralston, the 27-year-old mountaineer and outdoorsman, who set out on a weekend of adventure in remote southwest Utah, alone, and without telling anyone where he had gone. Now I am not saying that your running adventure is going to be as perilous a journey as Aron's was, but he would tell you to let someone know what your plan is so if something happens along the way, you have a backup who is looking for you. If you do not know who Aron Ralston is, rent the movie *127 Hours* starring James Franco.

Another recommendation is to take your cell phone with you when you run. In this day and age, there is no excuse for being without a means of reliable communication. Tuck your phone into your runner's pack or armband to have in case you turn an ankle, injure yourself if you trip and fall, sudden onset of chest pain, or you just plain get tired and cannot get home without collapsing. A cell phone is great to have if you are running in an unsavory part of town as well. You will be able to call for help from law enforcement if needed. You do not want to be at the mercy of any nuts out there who just love messing with runners. My encounters with people bothering me while running have been few but I have found that even though I may be tired in the middle of a run, I am in better shape than anyone like that giving me chase and I am able to quickly outdistance them while continuing to run. But in a pinch, I like to have my cell phone with me to call for help.

Headphones: Many folks like to listen to music while running. It takes their attention away from the physical exertion and steals their mind away, making the running more bearable I suppose. If you are a music lover and want to listen to something while running, I cannot object too vehemently if you are running in a park or on a trail with no traffic. It is not a good idea to do that around the neighborhood in proximity to traffic because you are limited to what you can see and not what you can see and hear. Using your senses is a great survival strategy. I suggest you employ them all.

One other reason for not piping music into your ears while running is it takes away from your ability to connect with your body. It keeps you from hearing the inner rhythm of your "machine" while you rev-up your engine. Being mindful of my breathing and heartbeat is something I look forward to during my runs, so I do not run with earphones.

Be Conscious: Besides making the attempt to be aware of your surroundings for signs of a dangerous situation, you must be aware of how your body parts are operating. You will encounter some aches and pains along the way as your fitness improves. Remember, "No pain, no gain." What I want to address here is the warning signs of an injury before it occurs. A turned ankle is obvious due to the acute nature of that injury. I am talking about listening to your body as you warm up, and as you progress in the run. Knowing what is normal as to the sensations you experience and what sensations are not normal is vital to your safety and success. You will not always be in tip-top shape for the workout regardless of your experience level. If something feels different, slow down or stop to check it out. Once you get into this running habit, you will want to do it religiously. It feels good. The thought of pulling back or taking an extra day to rest may not be in your plan while you prepare yourself for an event, but extra time stretching or resting between runs may save you from losing valuable training time.

I was about two weeks out from running in a half marathon and I was right on schedule as far as doing enough mileage. On my run the weekend before, I finished a nice ten-mile run at a suitable time and I was feeling great. It was mid-week, and I went out for a six-mile workout that was going to be a piece of cake. I stretched out as usual but had a tiny tingle in my left calf. I thought it was just a bit sore from the ten-miler I had just run, and I would need to just start slow and build my speed in the end. The tingle persisted past the point where I should have been warmed up completely, but it was not bad, so I continued. With about a half mile to go that tiny tingle turned into an excruciating pain that made me stop on a dime. The pain was so intense, I could hardly walk. I tried stretching it on the curb, and flexing out the muscles, but nothing was working. I had really done it and decided not to run at all until the day of the half marathon. I did all right during the event, but wondered how I could have done had I listened to my body and throttled back or not run at all that day that my calf felt strange. Remember: *"An ounce of prevention equals a pound of cure."*

Rules of the Road: If you have done your homework and choose a place like a park with a trail, you still must be careful out there. Just like when driving a car, there are rules to the road when running. Remember, unless you are out there at "zero-dark-thirty," you will be sharing the trail with others. There are bikers, walkers, runners, roller bladers, etc., all using what their tax dollars have bought. Generally speaking, the faster you go, the more you should watch out for others. But as you may figure, not everyone out there goes by the same rules, so, you should yield to the faster entity. Make it easy for bikers to go around you by staying to the side of the trail as much as possible. They should speak up and tell you of their approach by saying "bike on your left," or something like that. You should speak to slower traffic as well (walkers, mothers with baby strollers, etc.). It just makes sense to avoid a collision.

One of the other things I try to be courteous about is when I spit out water or blow my nose while running. Be aware of someone approaching from the rear. There is no better way to "meet" a new friend than by spitting or snorting on them. Some of you may not believe that blowing your nose on the run is something that you will have to do or even something that is possible. Believe me, once you start getting healthier, your body will start to get rid of phlegm and mucus from your lungs and sinuses. You cannot stop to blow it out, and if you do not blow it out, your airway will become constricted, making it hard to breathe. If you do not know how to clear your throat and spit out the gunk, you better practice.

The nose blowing technique is easy. Lay a finger aside your nostril, pressing it closed, and blow out through the other nostril with a slight head turn to that side to avoid having snot on your shirt. Be sure to look for approaching traffic from the rear on that side first. Repeat for the other nostril. This courtesy is especially important during a running event when perhaps thousands of other folks are running with you. Just remember to be aware of where you are and of others close to your space or passing by you. It just may be the thing that saves an injury or worse while you are out on the road training.

So, now we have our gear, a place to run, and all the safety advice we need. It is time to start doing it, right? Wrong! The next thing we need is a training plan.

Chapter 4: Plan for Training

In this chapter we will begin a discussion about the training itself. But before we start training, there is something we need to do first. Whether we are training for a marathon, half marathon, a 10K, or a Triathlon, we should have a training plan. The first step in making a plan is to decide what we are training for. My daughter chose the half marathon for my first challenge, but you will have to decide how far you want to go.

Let us start with the reason you might want to challenge yourself by choosing an event such as a marathon, half marathon, etc. to begin this program. Well, simply put, why would you go through the effort and stress of doing the running if you do not have some goal in mind? You do not have to run in an organized event, but it helps to have some sort of goal to shoot for. If you are not going to get out there with the crowd at a local 10K race or something like that, then you will have to set some sort of fitness goal to pull you forward in your new adventure. Some of you will like being able to run a mile or so and be satisfied with shaving off a few seconds each month from your favorite run. That is great. All you need to do now is run and monitor your time periodically as you improve your fitness.

For me there is nothing like setting a goal that will be challenging. In my opinion, a goal like this is measurable in terms of performance and is also defined by a time frame. For example, the two goals I set for my first half marathon were to finish in less than three hours, and to run the entire distance without stopping. These might not sound like very lofty goals, but you must remember, I was

55 years old and was, until recently, tipping the scale at over 300 lbs when I started this trek. I had about six weeks to prepare, which was not long enough to ease into it, so my first half marathon was agony at the end. However, I accomplished my goals by running 13.1 miles in 2:45:48, and I ran (or at least a reasonable facsimile of running) for the entire distance. I celebrated meeting the challenge, but I did not meet it with style. I crossed the finish line and was hurting so badly, I thought I would be crippled for weeks. I really hurt myself during that escapade and vowed to learn more about training for long-distance running events. I had to be smarter and better trained on the next one. In truth, that is when my training plan began. My desire here is to save you from putting yourself at risk like I did if you decide to do any competitive distance running. We will discuss the specific learning points a bit later. Suffice to say, I had a long way to go – in more ways than one.

So, when you have your idea of a goal in mind, you can start putting a training plan together. My rule of thumb for training is simple. Whatever the distance is that you want to train for, you should allow one week of training for each mile of the event you wish to run. This applies to your first or your second attempt at that particular event. After that, you can maintain a certain level of fitness between events and shorten your preparation time. For example, for a half marathon (13.1 miles), you should dedicate 12 - 13 weeks to train up to that level. Until you are in top shape for your age and for a certain level of intensity, I would not train less than half the number of weeks for each mile of any event after your first outing. So, plan for at least six training weeks for your second and subsequent half marathons.

The human body is an amazing machine, capable of doing incredible things if we treat it right. Maybe one of the most amazing things about the human body is that it will adjust to whatever gradual stress is put on it. In other words, our body will do what is asked of it. With increased resistance, or work, our bodies will get stronger, again, within certain "norms." With less resistance and less work, it will get weaker. So, another little truth I use regarding the training effort while preparing for an event is as follows:

The effort you put into training will be what your body gets used to. Whatever distance and speed you run in training will be what your body adjusts to, and you will most likely not run as well beyond that distance or at a faster speed.

So, for example, if your longest run in preparation for a 10K (6.2 miles) is only four miles – even if during your training period you run quite a few four-mile runs – during the 10K you will not be well prepared for the last 2.2 miles. Your muscle memory and your cardio-pulmonary capacity is set for an effort to carry you for four miles. Unless you do some intense interval training, which will be discussed later in this chapter, your body will "settle in" on the distance at which you train. Ideally, you should put in at least one or two 7 – 8 mile runs during your training period. That way your "wall" is beyond the 6.2-mile mark. Training for longer distances above the half marathon level requires different training regimens due to how our bodies store energy on which to run. For the average person in peak condition, the human body seems to run out of energy at about the 2-hour mark. Of course, there are those who push much farther than that on some of the eco-challenge type races, or ultra-triathlons, but that is in a whole different universe than the one I am talking about. For me, at least once during my 12-week work up, a run of about 13 – 15 miles two weeks prior to a half marathon seems to help me ease into the distance I am training for.

Always start out gradually with shorter runs in the first couple of weeks and increase your distances as you progress to the date of the event. You should do 3 – 4 runs per week with some cross training days sprinkled in to keep you from getting into a training rut. Always stretch well before you run, and you should have some days where you work on stretching and strengthening with no running at all. Plan for one relatively longer run one day each week. I do mine on Saturday mornings.

About half of your runs should be at least one-half to three-quarters of the distance you are training for and, as I mentioned above, try for one or two runs longer than your chosen event distance. So, if you are running a half marathon, half your runs will be 6 - 8 miles with two at 13 - 15 miles during the training period. You should at least be able to go for a 10-mile run before you attempt a half marathon. If you can do ten miles, then inspiration should help carry you the last 3.1 miles during the event. Your last "longest" run should come a week or more prior to the event with the last week as a taper down period with two days of no runs (and lots of stretching) just before the event. An example of a half marathon training schedule can be found at Hal Higdon's website (halhigdon.com).

Interval Training: One thing I learned from my study of this activity and from speaking with some professional runners, like Frank Shorter, Gold Medalist in the Marathon during the 1972 Olympic Games, is that you do not have the time to run increasingly longer distances to prepare for your planned run distance. I learned the best way to prepare for a Marathon, or longer run, is to conduct Interval Training. This type of work-out employs shorter distances run at faster speeds than normal for a section, or interval, of the run. The technique I used was to run around a quarter-mile track sprinting the straight leg and "coasting" at a slower pace around the curved portion of the track. In this way your body gets to experience "oxygen debt" without having to run to your "wall" which will be father out as you continue to train.

Running is only part of the training you need to consider if you want to seriously compete in any organized events. During a longer run, you will have to make sure you are well hydrated before, during and after the run. During an organized event, there will most likely be water/electrolyte stations at intervals (every couple of miles) along the event course. While training you will have to carry your own water (or whatever electrolyte liquid you want). You will also want to investigate carrying your own energy supplements to give your body the fuel it needs to keep going at a higher level. Otherwise, you will move at a slower and slower pace as you continue to run.

Unless you are a sponsored runner, you will have to carry your own energy supplements during the event as well. We will discuss these nutrient supplements later. Suffice to say, it is not just getting out there and running. You have to take care of yourself during the run if you want to finish strong. The following general information will help get you on your way:

Pace: Don't worry about how fast you run your regular workouts. Run at a comfortable pace. If you are training with a friend, the two of you should be able to carry on light conversation while running. If you cannot do that, you might be running too fast. If you wear a heart rate monitor, your target zone should be between 65 and 75 percent of your maximum heart rate according to your age. You can determine maximum heart rate by subtracting your age from 220.

Distance: The training schedule dictates workouts at distances, from 0.25 to 1.2 times the event distance. Do not worry about running precisely those distances, but you should come close.

Rest: Rest is as important a part of your training as the runs. It is imperative to let your body recover as you train. You will be better able to run the longer runs and limit your risk of injury if you rest the day before and the day after that run.

Long Runs: The key to getting ready to finish a long run is to progressively increase the distance of the long run each weekend. Over a period of 12 - 13 weeks, your weekly long run should increase by a mile or so each week. Your schedule may be set up so the long runs are done on Saturdays, but you can do them Sundays, or any other convenient day, as long as you are consistent. (See "Juggling," below.)

Cross-Train: What form of cross-training works best? It could be swimming, cycling, walking (see below), cross-country skiing, snowshoeing, or even some combination that could include strength training if you choose to do it on different days of the week than the indicated run days on your schedule. Feel free to throw in any aerobic activity that suits you. In fact, on one of the mid-week run days you may want to run or cross-train. What cross-training you select depends on your personal preference. But do not make the mistake of cross-training too vigorously. Cross-training days should be considered easy days that allow you to recover from the running you do during the rest of your week.

Walking: Walking is an excellent exercise that a lot of runners overlook in their training. I highly advocate using a walking break when needed. You should feel free to walk during your running workouts and events any time you feel tired or need to shift gears. When you go to the starting line for the event, do not be concerned whether you will run the entire distance; be more concerned that you finish! If that means walking during training or in the race, do it! An important note about resting during the event relating to pace is that, at some point, you may require slowing a bit to get your pulse under control. You can then speed back up to your personal best race speed to finish. If that means walking a few hundred yards, so be it. After you train for a while, you will be able to "throttle back" to a slower pace while continuing to run to get your heart rate back to an "elevated rest" level.

Interval training runs help to get you conditioned to throttle back and up during the run event. You may turn in a faster run time when you take a short "running rest break" when you are tired, than if you slug it out and run as fast as you can the entire distance. Slugging in out is what I did in my first half marathon, and I found myself going slower and slower as the run progressed. Walking at a brisk pace uphill gives you a rest at a time when you would be moving at a slower pace anyway while continuing to "run." The key is you will use more energy "running" under those conditions than you will while walking briskly at the same speed.

Stretching & Strengthening: The day following your long run day is the day on which I advise you to spend extra time stretching and, if you can, do some strength training too. This is a day of "rest" following your long run on the weekends, so do not overdo it. It is wise to stretch every day, particularly after you finish your run, but spend more time stretching on the day following your long run. Strength training could consist of push-ups, pull-ups, use of free weights or working out with various machines at a health club. Runners generally benefit if they combine light weights with a high number of repetitions, rather than pumping very heavy iron. I also suggest that you do strength training following your mid-week workouts; however, you can schedule strength training on any two convenient days.

Take Your Time: Does the designated number of weeks for your event progression seem too tough? Do you have more than that number of weeks before your selected event? Lengthen the schedule; take as many weeks as you need to prepare. You can even repeat the week just completed before moving up to the next level. Do not be afraid to insert "step back" weeks, where you actually cut your distance every second or third week to gather forces for the next push forward.

Racing: It is not obligatory, but you might want to run a 5K or 10K race to see how you are doing - and to experience a road race if you have not run one before. You will be able to use your run times to predict your finishing time in the chosen event and get acquainted with what pace you may want to run that race. In training for a half marathon, I suggest a 5K race at the half-way point in your training schedule and a 10K race at the three-quarter mark.

Juggling: Don't be afraid to juggle the workouts from day to day and week to week. If you have an important business meeting on Thursday when you normally do your long run, do that workout on Wednesday instead. If your family is going to be on vacation during one of your training weeks when you will have more or less time to train, adjust the schedule accordingly. If you are consistent with your training, the overall details will not matter. Just be sure to get the right amount of work in each week.

Cheating: There really is no cheating; either you can do the distance or not. If you find yourself a little behind the scheduled run distances, do not worry, you can repeat a week to get to a certain level before pushing yourself to meet the distance prescribed. You can also swap days for particular runs to accommodate a schedule change as mentioned above. On the other hand, if you feel good and want to go a little farther than the schedule calls for, then let yourself go. If you are sticking with the scheduled number of runs per week at the prescribed distances, most likely you will be in great shape for the upcoming event.

To get the best out of the time you put into any program, be consistent. Your body will respond and let you know what is working and what is not. Once you are in the groove, you will miss the training if you do not go out a day or two during any week. Just like anything else, you will be forming a new habit, and once you latch on, it becomes a part of you. Find your level of fitness and enjoyment, then go with it, whatever that level is. Setting a mileage goal for yourself will help keep you in the game. Have fun but make a serious attempt to improve. The dividends will be paid in years to come – believe it.

As for me, my training has paid off in my performance during running events. In my second half marathon, I was able to finish a much tougher course with much less trauma to my body. Although I ran it in about the same time, I was not hurting at all when the finish line crossed me. I was contending with a small pull in my calf that undoubtedly slowed me down a bit, but I still had a decent run. In my third run I shaved off 15 minutes from the previous time, with a similar improvement for my fourth run in my first year of running half marathons.

I was getting faster gradually and set my goal to attain a sub-2-hour half marathon time in my second year of running. I have not had to kill myself so far in advancing toward that goal. The operative word here is "gradual." You do not have to set any records or try to win a professional contract, just give it a little consistency and you will feel, look, and be better.

It can give you a sense of satisfaction to be doing this type of activity in your fifties and sixties. During my first half marathon, I was amazed at the number of folks that were my age or older. I will tell you about one of them later in Chapter 8. It was clear to me that this was an activity that I could participate in for years to come with a little training. Even though I was dead tired, I experienced a real sense of accomplishment. Once you do one of these runs, you will never go back to your old ways. If someone had told me years ago that I would be running half marathons, I would have laughed myself silly. But now it is a part of me, and I will do it for years to come. Doing this type of running has allowed me to continue to do other outdoor activities like backpacking and kayaking that I had given up on due to my poor physical condition

- they just ceased to be enjoyable any longer. But now I have a new lease on life.

In the next chapter I will discuss some things about how you can manage the work you have set before yourself. As I mentioned previously, you will be changing and adjusting as you do this work. And just like when you go through the changes in diet, your body will protest, in its own way. Since you want this endeavor to be as enjoyable as possible, you will need some tricks of the trade, so-to-speak, that will help keep you on track and give you some tools to measure your progress. See you in Chapter 5.

Chapter 5: Turning On and Tuning In

Even though I was not necessarily a "runner," I thought that I could use the challenge of getting ready for a half marathon, and the specter of public humiliation if I could not finish, to motivate myself to get in shape. If you are not a runner, you can use most of the training principles I discuss in whatever activity that suits you. The advantage of using long-distance running as a training tool is that you do not need an expensive gym membership, or any type of sophisticated equipment. As I mentioned before, you just need a decent pair of shoes and the great outdoors in which to run. And running in half marathons presents opportunities to visit different areas of the country and participate with thousands of fellow running enthusiasts. I am certainly grateful for the opportunity to share something like this with my adult daughters. Besides all that, I feel younger each year I do this and, of course, Mom stopped telling me I was "fat."

In this chapter we are going to talk about what it is for which we are shooting; turning onto and preparing for the changes that will take place as we start to exercise regularly. Since I have formed a new habit, I feel as if I am cheating myself when I miss a workout. And that is true, for the most part, I am cheating myself, but I do not beat myself up about it. I just enjoy the next run all the more. Besides, even if I miss a run now and again, I am doing vastly more exercise in a week than I did in a year prior to starting my running workouts. I find that my self-esteem is elevated just thinking about what I can do now compared to a relatively brief time ago.

We are also going to talk about "tuning in" with our body's vibrations. Once you tune into the natural rhythms inside you, the joy of the activity will take over and you will seemingly glide through your workouts. When you attain just a slight improvement in your physical condition, hearing the mantra of your heart beating and of your breathing will have a hypnotic effect on your consciousness. We will also talk about being in tune with your body from a musculoskeletal point of view. Being aware of how your muscles feel and the signals they give you is important if you expect to enjoy this activity for longer than a few runs. Lastly, we will see how this information plugs into our performance while training and in the actual running event.

In talking about "turning on," we need to discuss habits and how we as humans form and change our habits. From a purely psychological point of view, the behaviors that we repeat regularly become habits. Put another way, our repeated behaviors become routines which tend to occur subconsciously.[17] [18] Because a person does not engage in self-analysis when undertaking routine tasks, the routine behavior often goes unnoticed.[19] Habituation is an extremely simple form of learning, in which a human, after a period of exposure to a stimulus, stops responding to that stimulus in varied manners.[20] Habits sometimes become compulsory. Just as sitting around and becoming a couch potato requires repeated behavior, becoming regularly active with a workout routine will become a

---

[17] Butler, Gillian; Hope, Tony. *Managing Your Mind: The mental fitness guide.* Oxford Paperbacks, 1995

[18] Definition of *Habit. Merriam Webster Dictionary.* Retrieved on August 29, 2008

[19] Definition of *Habituation. Merriam Webster Dictionary.* Retrieved on August 29, 2008

[20] "Habituation." Animalbehavioronline.com.

habit when repeated. The paradox in this equation is we must consciously repeat the routine of working out for long enough until the desire to repeat that action becomes a part of our subconscious mind.

Why do you want to make this a subconscious habit? Because once it is habit with you to do your workouts, the longer you will stick with it. In the last chapter we talked about planning your training. One of the big reasons for planning is for you to feel in control of your activity and another is to give you a sense of accomplishment when you complete the training in your plan. The idea of making a habit of this is two-fold as well. First, you will feel better and gain a level of health that you did not know you could reach. Secondly, forming this habit will keep you going when all else fails. In essence, you will learn to love it.

Tuning in is the real reward in this for me. Once I am out on the road or trail and breaking a sweat, I can let the entire world go. Although I do my morning and evening meditations at home, there is nothing like the rhythm of the run to bring out some great meditative effects. And just as you must discipline yourself to stay in your meditative state in the quiet of your favorite room or place, you must train for this meditative state as well.

When I start my runs, I usually push myself for a while before I can relax and lean into the running. It takes at least a half mile before I am loosened up, even though I stretch thoroughly before each run. During that first half mile or so, I concentrate on getting my breathing coordinated with my running rhythm. My heart will pick up the pace as the demand for oxygen increases. I do not have to think about speeding up my heart rate, my autonomic nervous system takes care of that for me. My respiratory system will naturally speed up in accordance with the demand as well. With some practice, I have been able to affect my heart rate during quiet meditation, but on the run, I let my heartbeat as it will. Controlling your respiration on the run is much easier and, as it turns out, quite necessary if you intend to run for any significant distance.

The tendency for the untrained runner is to hyperventilate when the stress of running begins. As I take a breath in, I am drawing the needed oxygen into my lungs to burn the glucose I have stored. As I breathe out, my body gets rid of carbon dioxide, a byproduct from the reaction of oxygen and glucose that occurs as I exercise. My respiratory system is constantly working to keep the proper amount of oxygen in the hard-working muscles. To do this it detects the level of carbon dioxide through a system of neuro-chemical receptors that are found in the bloodstream. In normal breathing both the frequency and the depth of the breath are controlled by this system. During hyperventilation, the lungs are exhaling more carbon dioxide than is being produced through exercise. The low carbon dioxide level in the bloodstream causes the blood vessels to constrict which decreases the ability to transport oxygen to all parts of the body. The cycle continues as the breathing speeds up to get more oxygen into the system to supply the deprived muscles that are working so hard.

Hyperventilation is the body's attempt to process more oxygen so the muscles can do more work.[21]

---

[21] Martin, Elizabeth A (ed.) (2003). *Oxford concise medical dictionary* (6th ed.w. corrections & new cover). Oxford University Press. p. 334. ISBN 10:0-19-60753

Hyperventilation occurs when a person exercises over their VO2 max, the point when the body is unable to transform oxygen into energy beyond a certain level. Our VO2 max is the maximum ability for our bodies to consume oxygen. Heredity has a great deal to do with your VO2 max. While we can improve our VO2 max level, there is only so much we can do to increase that ability due to our genetics.[22]

If you are hyperventilating while running, slow down and catch your breath. As mentioned earlier, you should be able to carry on light conversation while running or at least be able to control your breathing. This will help you stay safely out of the hyperventilation range.[23] [24]

To prevent going into hyper-ventilation, I work on controlling my breathing while running. The best way I know to control my breath is to match my breathing pace with my foot strike pace. I breathe in and out each time my left foot strikes the ground. That is, I begin breathing in when my left foot hits the ground and continue that breath until my left foot hits the ground again when the exhale begins (see Diagram 1 on the next page). In essence, this is a two-count breathing technique. Breathing this way allows for a sufficient volume of air exchange. Use this technique for running on level ground or when

---

[22] "Arteriovenous oxygen difference". *Sports Medicine, Sports Science and Kinesiology*. Net Industries and its Licensors.011.http://sports.jrank.org/pages /5973/arteriovenous-oxygen-difference.html

[23] Gardner W (April 2000). "Orthostatic increase of respiratory gas exchange in hyperventilation syndrome". *Thorax* 55 (4): 2579.doi:10.1136/thorax.55.4.257. PMC1745726. PMID10722762. http://www.pubmedcentral.nih.gov /articlerender.fcgi?tool=pmcentrez&artid=1745726.

[24] http://www.yourdictionary.com Hyperventilation Citing: The American Heritage®

you are starting your run before settling into your pace and relaxing your stride.

DIAGRAM 1

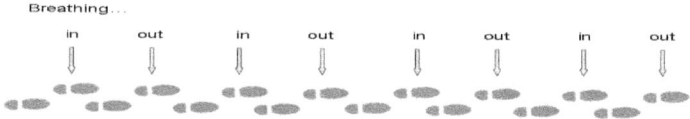

Keeping a steady pace and breath control is important when running long distances if you want to have a respectable time during a run or race. When the demand for oxygen in the body increases due to increased effort, your breath pace should increase too. For example, while running uphill you will either slow down your running pace and keep the same breath pace or keep the same run pace and increase your breath pace to match the demand of the increased work of climbing the hill. My technique for keeping my run pace on a climb is to consciously quicken my breath pace to get more breaths in with the same number of strides.

Diagram 2 on the next page shows how my breathing matches up with my run pace as I hit an incline during a run. You can see that you will get one more breath in the same number of steps using that technique. Obviously, you will need to quicken the exchange from exhale to inhale to get a full breath. This new breath pace creates a new rhythm and seems to help me concentrate on my breathing instead of the climb.

Once the hill has been conquered and the demand for an increased level of oxygen subsides, getting back to your normal running breath pace is crucial to your success in finishing the run. After you get into better condition, controlling your breathing will become second nature. You will fall into that rhythm and relax into the run after tuning in on your natural pace.

DIAGRAM 2

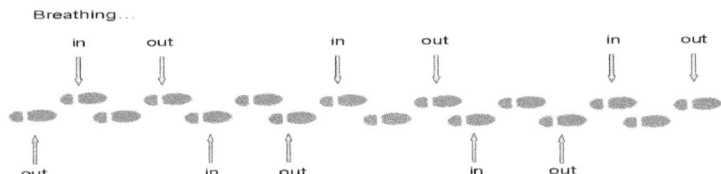

I need to say just a few more words about breathing. It is a popular myth that you should breathe in through your nose and out through your mouth. The amount of air able to be delivered through the nose is inadequate for the oxygen demands on your body while running. As you breathe in you should allow air to enter through both nose and mouth. This will give you the maximum available intake and give your muscles more needed oxygen to keep moving. Also, be sure that you are breathing from your diaphragm, or belly, and not your chest. Chest breathing is too shallow and will not give you enough air with each breath inhaled. Exhale through the mouth and focus on exhaling fully to expel as much carbon dioxide as possible with each breath. This will also help you inhale more deeply.

I mentioned before that you should be able to make light conversation while running. If you feel out of breath, slow down or stop until your breathing is under control. I have been advised by experienced runners to take three-foot strikes for each inhale and three for the exhale which looks like Diagram 3 below.

DIAGRAM 3

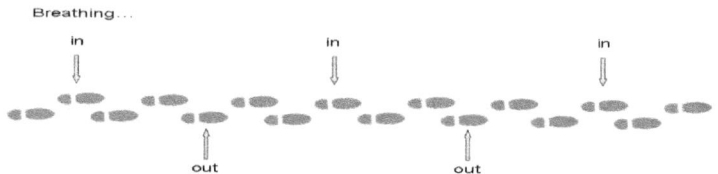

The two steps per breath pace I shared earlier is what worked for me when I began to run. Now I usually employ a three-step breathing rhythm when I am running downhill or after I have really settled into a run on level ground. You should strive to take as many strides per full breath as possible while running. In other words, if you can supply your body with adequate oxygen while taking more strides per breath, then all the better for you. You will necessarily be in better shape when you can use this breath pace. Do your own experimentation and see what works for you. If you are relaxed during the run, breathing should take care of itself. Do not try to outsmart your body.

Tuning into your musculoskeletal system is as important as being in touch with your cardiopulmonary system. As I said, the human body is an amazing machine. It can endure some intense stress and recover to repeat the performance when it is well cared for. The idea of training the human body to perform at increasingly higher levels athletically must be tempered with restraint in the knowledge of how much it can take at any one time. Just as in any mechanical apparatus there are limits to what we can put our bodies through. For example, every pilot knows that there are four types of limits that they can induce on the airframe they fly.

The Load Limit: defined as the maximum load a structure, in this case the airframe, can safely carry without damage. Next is the Damage Limit which is defined as a load greater than the Load Limit where structural damage *may* occur, however slight. The structure will flex, shortening the life of the airframe. The Ultimate Limit is next defined as a load under which structural damage *will* occur. In other words, the airframe will bend, and the aircraft will need repairing. The Failure Limit is next and is defined as a load that will produce failure of the airframe. Operations beyond this limit will produce a catastrophic failure from which the airframe cannot recover. This is where the wings fall off or something like that. Important safety tip: Do not fly beyond the Failure Limit.[25]

So, how does all this information apply to the human body? Well, a damaged airframe can be repaired by a mechanic after a careless pilot flies it beyond the structural limitation. But it cannot necessarily grow stronger in the process of the "work out," or stress sustained while flying. Even if the aircraft is never flown beyond the load limit, it

---

[25] Structural Limits, from http://www.tpub.com/content/aviation2/P-1231/P-12310035.htm

will weaken over time. Every airplane has a structural lifetime after which it needs to be retired. However, our bodies can grow stronger, within certain norms, over time with work or stress applied to them.

What's more is the fact that our bodies always tell us when we are overstressing it. We will get sore and tired. The feeling of growing muscles does not have to be painful, but we will feel it after a workout. For the beginner, the "damage limit" is much lower than for the intermediate or advanced athlete. So, we must respect our bodies as we whip them into shape, and you do not need an expert to tell you how much you can take. Your body will certainly let you know – listen to it. This is especially important after you have gained some strength and conditioning. Listening to your body can save you a great deal of pain and keep you on the road instead of convalescing. Each time you are required to lay off due to a pull, tear, or some form of overworked body part, you regress in the training program. It is a shame to waste all the good work done in preparation for an event because of something preventable.

The key to success here is to become more conscious about what you are doing to yourself. We hopefully have transitioned from stuffing ourselves and sitting on our "keisters," to eating well and improving our physical condition to start really enjoying life. There is another component of all this that I will discuss more thoroughly in Chapter 9. For now, I will only mention that we, as human beings, have a huge energetic component to our existence here on earth. Some would argue that we are all energy. I do not know to what degree that is true, however, I can tell you that there is something going on besides biology and psychology.

A good detective would say, "There's something more here than meets the eye," which I interpret as meaning there is more to it than what we see in front of our eyes. I believe there is something going on behind the scenes to account for as well. Unfortunately, that sort of logic does not come from what everyone is thinking. Put another way, we have all heard a doubting Thomas say, "I'll believe it when I see it," when something does not meet with their interpretation of the Universe. They are stuck in needing the Universe to show them before they know what is so. But what is true for me is just the opposite statement, "I'll see it when I believe it."

Changing my life through a certain activity taught me one immutable truth about our world; we are each responsible for how we perceive our existence. The discovery by 15th century Europeans that our planet was spherical instead of flat certainly changed the knowledge base in the old world. But more significant than that is the fact that it changed perceptions of the Earth and utilizing that viewpoint, new worlds were discovered. It is apparent that we are more than muscle and blood. I will attempt to tell the story later in the book of how I found my spiritual essence. Discovering your spiritual self will help you "tune in and turn on" before you "tap out!"

In the next chapter we will discuss a few specific maladies associated with this activity. I will suggest some "homemade" cures and some preventative measures to help you cope with the stress that you are going to undergo. I hope you got the point that taking on this activity does not have to be a Herculean task. Be smart and manage the pain down to a tolerable minimum to survive to a level where you will start to enjoy this. Happy running!

Chapter 6: Aches and Pains

♫ Nobody knows the trouble I've seen; nobody knows my sorrow. ♫

When we start to hit the road, we will encounter some rough spots in our journey. There will be the inevitable aches and pains associated with the increasing stress we will experience. Call them growing pains. What I want to address in this chapter are the "normal" or "common" troubles that plague all runners and a few things that will affect certain "body types."

I want to be clear here and reiterate that I am not a healthcare professional by any standard. I do not even play one on television. The information to be shared in this chapter is not intended to replace information received by a healthcare professional pertaining to an injury you have sustained. In fact, the conditions I describe herein may sound like what you are experiencing, but it is up to you to determine whether what you have encountered rises to a level that needs to be addressed by an expert or by the information I am imparting. My purpose is to give you some information to negotiate minor aches and pains to keep you going. My guidance here does not pertain to injuries. The difference between "minor aches and pains" and "injury" is that an injury will need the attention of a healthcare professional.

Before we jump into the pit of despair with the possible aches and pains associated with this adventure, let us talk about prevention. The best way to keep on the healthy side of this is to properly warm up and stretch out before and after every run – every single run!

Cold muscles are easily injured. Warm them up with some low-impact, basic rhythmic movements like walking or light jogging in place. Jumping jacks are a terrific way to warm up the entire body to including your core and arms as well as your legs. Take about 5 minutes to get warm before moving to your stretching routine.

Stretching is especially important and will provide some benefits beyond getting ready to exercise. When properly done, stretching increases flexibility and balance which is essential for athletic activity. It also improves posture and alignment which helps body mechanics. Circulation will also increase the more you stretch. The relief of aches and pains is aided by stretching and stress is released with each repetition of the stretching motion. Along with all these added benefits, our main objective in stretching is to prevent injury while exercising. The old saying, *"An ounce of prevention is worth a pound of cure"* is certainly true when it comes to stretching before physical activity.

While stretching, remember to move slowly and do not bounce. You want to gradually apply tension to the muscle group you are stretching without causing pain. If it hurts, back off and build your flexibility over time. Hold the position at a maximum stretch without pain for 30 to 60 seconds. Repeat the stretch as necessary until you feel relaxed in that position. Always breathe while stretching. The idea is to relax. Holding your breath will increase the tension in your body. Remember, this should feel good.

The actual stretches you do are up to you. Just be sure to stretch all the areas necessary to warm and prepare the muscles you will be using for the work to come. I like to do the following stretches before I go for a run. If, like most of us, you had gym class in high school, you have done these stretches before:

Hurdler's Stretch: in a seated position on the ground with one leg straight in front of you (back of the knee on the ground) and the other pulled back and to the side of you (like the position a hurdler is in when clearing the hurdle), lean the torso forward, back straight, until the tension is felt. Ideally, you will eventually be able to touch your forehead to your straightened knee. A modification of this position is with the back leg bent in front of you placing the bottom of the foot on the inside of the straight leg's knee. Switch and stretch both sides.

Spine Twist: still seated on the ground with both legs in front of you, bend one leg or the other placing the foot on the outside of the opposite leg touching your ankle to the knee. Then place your opposite elbow on the outside of the bent knee and press to twist your torso with your other arm behind you for support. Remember to keep your back straight to get the best out of this stretch without hurting yourself. Switch and stretch both sides.

Quadriceps Stretch: in a standing position near a wall or post for balance, bend your knee lifting your foot up behind you while reaching back to grasp your toe. Apply slight pressure stretching the quad muscles by pulling your heal closer to your buttocks. For extra stretch you can extend the bent knee back behind you. Be careful not to overstretch it. Switch and stretch both sides.

Lunge: in a standing position take a step forward with either leg placing that foot about two feet in front of the other. Slowly lunge forward keeping the back leg straight with the heal on the ground. Keep the torso upright and the back straight as well. Switch and stretch both sides.

Calf Stretch: stand near a wall or a fence extending your arms and pushing against it as if you were pushing it over. With one leg extended behind you and the other under you for balance, slowly stretch the calf on the straight leg, then switch legs and stretch again. By arching your back in this position and pressing forward with your hips, you can stretch the quadriceps and the torso as well. You can even put both legs back and lean into the wall stretching both calves at once. Relax each calf and do not allow them to flex or tighten during this stretch.

Side and Shoulder Stretch: while sitting or standing, extend either arm across and in front of your chest. Place your other forearm in a position behind the elbow of that arm. Pull the outstretched arm stretching the shoulder and side of the torso. Be sure to stretch the lat muscles when pulling the arm across your chest. Switch and stretch both sides. This is a good one to keep from having those "stitches" in your side as you run.

Now let us look at the bothersome little tweaks that seem to hamper our running fun.

Sore Muscles: When you up your game physically, you are bound to develop some soreness in your leg muscles. Even if you take it slowly, you will have some soreness. Let me define soreness a bit for the purpose of differentiating some of the conditions common to initiating or overdoing this activity. When I say "soreness" what I am talking about is discomfort, not pain necessarily, in your muscles due to over working them (and doing anything after sitting around for years is over working). It was thought that sore muscles are a result of a build-up of lactic acid in the muscle tissue, but the lactic acid is usually washed out within 30 to 60 minutes of the workout. Currently, the dominant theory is that when you exercise, even moderately, you cause a small amount of damage to the muscle fibers. The damaged muscle becomes swollen and sore. Chemicals are released from the damaged muscles which irritate nerve endings causing discomfort. There is also an increase in blood flow from increased activity of the muscle, causing tissues to swell producing pressure that stimulates pain receptors.[26] Your muscles will grow stronger as they repair themselves.

As a function of aging, our muscle tissue is less elastic so we will experience soreness more quickly and more intensely, and from less activity, than in our youth. Moving sore muscles will help return them to a more normal state. Stretching after the run will help alleviate soreness, but time is your best ally here. After you get used to working those muscles, you will not experience long-term soreness like when you begin your running routine. Drinking plenty of water or your favorite electrolyte drink will help too. For short-term relief there are topical ointments (sports balms, etc.) that relieve some of the pain. You can also take a hot bath or sit in a Jacuzzi to relieve the pain a bit, or you can sit in the sauna, but stretching out those painful muscles works best.

Sprains and Strains: What is the difference between a sprain and a strain? A sprain is a tear in the ligaments that are attached to the ends of bones. Ankles, knees, and wrists are all vulnerable to spraining. A strain is an

---

[26] Burke, E. Ph.D. Soreness - It's Not About the Lactic Acid: Why You're Still Sore After Yesterday's Ride, from http://www.active.com/mountainbiking /Articles/It_s_not_about_the_lactic_acid_Why_you_re_still_sore_after yesterday_s_ride.ht

overstretching of the muscles or tendons (the connective tissue between the muscle and the bone) that may result in a tear. If you experience an acute pain in a joint or in a muscle, see a healthcare professional. Treatment will vary depending on the severity of the sprain or strain. If you sustain either of these injuries, the first aid treatment is to use the "RICE" method which is Rest, Ice, Compress, Elevate. The "Rest" step is obvious. Stop running and let the healing begin. "Ice' is also obvious. Icing in the initial stages of the injury is important for a quicker recovery. Do not put heat on the area for at least 24 hours after the injury. "Compress" means to wrap the area with an elastic bandage to control swelling. If you sprain your ankle, it is advisable to keep the shoe on until you can wrap it or get medical help. "Elevate" by raising the injured part of your body higher than it normally would be, preferably in a position level with the heart, to keep the blood from pooling in that area.

Unless you can get to a healthcare facility right away, you should use the RICE method to control the swelling and ease the pain. But you need to get professional help for these types of injuries. The good news is, the better condition you are in, the less the risk of these types of injuries. Returning to activity after an injury of this type must be done gradually. Tune in and listen to your body's response to the intensity of the workout when you return.

Shin Splints (Medial Tibial Stress Syndrome MTSS): One of the most common conditions in runners is the occurrence of shin splints. This condition is the result of an injury to the posterior peroneal tendon and adjacent tissue in the front of the lower leg usually from running on hard surfaces. For the hard-core runner, taping the shin can allow for continued training, but I recommend a treatment of rest. Use the RICE method and continue to stretch while recovering. Once the pain of shin splints is bearable, try to lightly exercise your lower front leg by "air writing" the A B Cs with your toes while sitting before doing the Hurdler's Stretch and the Spine Twist. Doing this before you get shin splints is a great preventive measure.

Plantar Fasciitis: This is a painful injury of the tendon that runs from the heel to the front of the foot under the arch. Overstretching of the Plantar Fascia or Arch Tendon causes pain at the attach point of the tendon to the heel. This condition is usually caused by overly tight calf muscles. The tight calves lead to prolonged or high velocity pronation of the foot.[27] In other words, while running, when your foot rolls inward unnaturally, it stretches the tendon under the arch more than usual causing pain on the inside bottom of the heel. This injury will be more painful the morning after running when the tendon has tightened up over night. Rest is the only real cure. Taping the arch to support it and relieve the pressure has been found to help along with cold treatment of the area to reduce the inflammation.

Knee Pain: Patellofemoral Pain Syndrome is one cause of knee pain and is a fancy term for a sore kneecap or, more accurately, the tendons holding the patella.[28] This usually occurs from an anatomical misalignment problem that is best addressed by a qualified professional bio-mechanist or podiatrist. Suffice to say that knee joint pain may occur

---

[27] CommentActive.com plantar fasciitis, from http://www.distancerunning-tips.com/running-and-foot-pain.html

[28] Sports Injuries – top 5 running injuries, from http://www.podiatrym.com/cme/Apr08CME.df

because the muscles above the knee (the quadriceps) are too weak to properly move and align the knee while running. Proper strengthening exercises may be the ticket but get a professional opinion before trying to fix this type of condition by yourself.

As discussed in Chapter 2, if you have prolonged pronation (inward roll of the ankle) or supination (outward roll of the ankle), you also may feel some discomfort or pain in the knee. This misalignment in or out can translate to the medial (inner) or lateral (outer) part of the knee respectively being unduly stressed at that point, which overstretches the ligaments. This can further translate to the hip joint causing discomfort there as well. Knee pain can easily be corrected most of the time using an orthotic insert that rolls the ankle to a neutral and more stable position relieving the stress and pain that follows. Do not wing it and guess what will work. Be sure to get expert advice if this occurs to you.

Stress Fractures: This term is the common reference to what is known as Repetitive Stress Injury (RSI). The stress of running long distances puts great tension and compression on the bones of the lower extremities. Similar to the tiny tears in the muscles when overstressed, the bones of the human body will receive "micro-damage" that occurs faster than can be healed. Although not a fracture at all, stress fractures refer to the massive micro-damage built up by repetitive action. The tibia, metatarsals, and the calcaneus in the lower leg are most affected by RSI.[29]

Blisters: Blisters are small pockets of fluid in the upper layers of the skin caused by rubbing. Since we will ensure

---

[29] Ibid.

that our shoes fit properly, we should not have any trouble with blisters, right? That is the best preventive measure – well-fitting shoes. Even so, we may experience friction between the toes while running longer distances. Usually, blisters form more easily on wet skin. On a long run, your feet will sweat, and your socks will be soaked. I always put some petroleum jelly on (and in between) my toes, and around my heel to minimize the friction in those spots. It works well as I have yet to get a blister while running when I slather my feet up with the magic gel.

If you do get blisters, what is the best way to treat them? There is the ongoing battle of whether to lance or "pop" them or not. Our skin is a great defensive organ against all sorts of nasty things out there. Opening the skin by lancing a blister may give an opening to bacteria or some other biotic nemesis causing infection. Some say, "Pop that blister," and others say, "No!" I have a hybrid position. If they are small, leave them alone and cover them with an adhesive bandage like moleskin, which can be found at the local drug store. If they are large, with lots of fluid, lance it under as sterile a condition as you can make and, again, cover it with moleskin. Here are the steps to a clean and successful blister popping party.

1. Wash your hands and the blister with soap and warm water.

2. Swab the blister with iodine or rubbing alcohol.

3. Sterilize a clean, sharp needle by wiping it with rubbing alcohol.

4. Use the needle to puncture the blister. Aim for several spots near the blister's edge. Let the

fluid drain but leave the overlying skin in place.

5. Apply an antibiotic ointment to the blister and cover with a bandage or gauze pad (if you are running soon, cover with moleskin).

6. Cut away all the dead skin after several days, using tweezers and scissors sterilized with rubbing alcohol. Apply some more antibiotic ointment and a bandage.

7. Call your doctor if you see signs of infection around a blister — pus, redness, pain, or warm skin.[30]

Black Toenails: Black toenails are common among runners, especially those training for long-distance races. After some long runs, the toenails, especially on the big toe, become bruised and will eventually blacken due to bleeding under the nail. When training for a marathon, or doing a lot of downhill running, the toes are constantly rubbing up against the front of the shoes. Running in warmer weather will increase the likelihood of black toenails because the feet swell more when it is hot, causing greater toe to shoe contact. The constant rubbing of your toe against the front of your shoe produces a blood blister that forms under the nail. Since the blister cannot be easily drained, the healing takes a lot longer.

To help prevent black toenails, make sure that you are wearing the correct running shoe size as discussed in Chapter 2. Keep your toenails trimmed regularly, and

---

[30] **By Stephen Pribut, DPM Blisters, from** http://www.mayoclinic.com/health /first-aid-blisters/WL00008

make sure to keep your feet dry for as long as possible, especially during your long runs. Be sure to wear socks that wick sweat away from the foot. Cotton is not recommended. Try lacing your shoes tighter along the front if you are doing a lot of downhill running.

Once you have a black toenail, it is best to leave it alone, as long as the pain is manageable. The pain is usually the worst on the first day and then lessens each day after. The damaged part of the nail is gradually pushed off, and a new nail will replace it. Do not force the old nail off; it will fall off on its own. If at any point you notice redness and infection, see a healthcare professional.[31]

If you take it easy, and care for yourself along the way, most of what we discussed here will not come up for you. As you get stronger and more fit, you will naturally avoid these types of injuries. But if you fall victim to one or two of these, please take caution in the way you treat them. It is better to lay off for a while to recover completely, even if you lose the physical conditioning you attained, than to try to run through the hurt and making things worse. Sometimes it takes twice as long, or longer, to recover if you go back too soon. See a healthcare professional about anything you feel is not right with your body.

Well, we have talked about all the preliminary issues. Now let us get into the "fun stuff." It is about time for our first real running event.

---

[31] Black Toenail information from http://running.about.com/od/common runninginjuries /p/blacktoenail.htm

Chapter 7: Your First Running Event

So, you have changed your diet, bought the necessary gear, formed a plan, trained hard, tuned into your body, cared for your wounds. Now what? If you think you are ready, it is time for your first real running event – and believe me, if you have done all that, you are ready!

Depending on what races in which you are thinking of participating (I like to call them runs because I do not race anyone but myself), most likely there are a number of events close to you that offer an opportunity to excel. You will be able to find information about running events at your local sporting goods store or health club, but the best way to find the information you need is by using the greatest tool ever devised by humankind, the Internet. Just type "running events" into Google or any search engine on the Internet to find information on 5K through marathon events that are within driving distance. You will even find out about ultra marathons, trail runs, kids runs and running camps. As you get more in tune with this type of activity, you may branch out and seek events in different areas of the country, presenting an opportunity to visit a new town in which to have fun while you run.

There is usually a fee for participating as the support for putting on these types of events does require funding, even when volunteer help is enlisted. There are many runs that raise money for charity or for medical research, so you can do something worthwhile with your time and money while improving your health. There are usually events around holidays as well, such as the various "Turkey Trots" on Thanksgiving weekend. The big weekends for events are Memorial Day and Labor Day like many socially oriented events, but you will be able to find a run every weekend somewhere in the country. There are even memorial runs of varying distances in every area of the United States every month of the year as well. One of the more notable memorial runs is Pat's Run in Tempe, Arizona in honor of the fallen hero of the war in Afghanistan, Pat Tillman. The Pat Tillman Foundation puts the run on in April every year around the time of Pat's birthday. I do not usually endorse any runs, and I am not pushing for Pat's Run, but I do like the idea of finding something like that to participate in and that one is a good one.

It is important to select a run distance that you are going to be able to finish. Do not worry about setting an Olympic record; just finish. If you started this adventure in terrible shape, and your mile and a half time is somewhere around 30 minutes, do not despair, you will be able to finish a 5K run, or 3.1 miles, in fine time. Just have fun. If you have spent at least six weeks running three times a week, you should have no problems. If you are in better shape, you can go the distance and pick something a bit more challenging. My formula for selecting a distance to run for beginners is to take whatever distance you have trained up to, let us say five miles, and multiply it by 1.3 to give you the distance for which you should try. So, five miles times a factor of 1.3 gives you 6.5 miles. You should easily be able to run a 10K road race which is 6.2 miles.

Now, you have researched the race in which you want to participate and at a distance and location that suits you. What's next? Well, you should sign up as early as possible for the event. I find that when I am signed up for a road race well in advance, I can more easily plan around it with other life events instead of trying to squeeze it in, having to rearrange plans I have already made. The real reason for me to schedule an event in advance is that it gives me more motivation to get out and do my runs. Having something to shoot for is great for helping me put my all into anything I do. In Chapter 10 I will share with you some of the things I do in helping to plan for and execute my run preparation schedule.

In most every run you will be issued a race number when you register. I know of none that do not do this. The larger the run event is, the bigger the "perks." In the larger running events, marathons, and half marathons, you pay more to run, but you get a bit more too. Besides, most of the bigger events support charity organizations as well. Here is a list of things to help you know what to expect and what to do for the big event:

Health & Fitness Exposition: Usually one or two days prior to the road race the big events feature a sports expo, usually held in a nearby convention center, which includes all sorts of new products offered by vendors large and small. The latest gear for the avid runner from shoes to clothing to energy drinks (and more) can be found there. The biggest events have corporate sponsorship and receive big advertising attention. Sometimes you will find guest speakers and famous athletes at these event expos. Do your homework before going and take with you something you may want to have autographed such as a picture of the athlete or a piece of running gear. I once got Frank Shorter to sign my race number, and Jim Ryan, the first American to run a sub four-minute mile, to autograph one of his books I brought. They each gave the audience some useful information about the sport of running during their time on the guest podium. After their talks I found both gentlemen to be very accessible and willing to speak with me personally. It was quite a thrill for me and motivating for the run the next day to be sure. Go to the expo, it is worth the time.

Packet Pick-up: At the expo, or sometime before the day of the race, you should be able to pick up your packet for the race. If there is no expo or prior pick-up time, get to the event early on race day to get your number and prepare for the race. At a minimum, the packet will include your number bib, a final information sheet, and a liability disclaimer to sign. The bigger events will allow you to download this information and legal paperwork well prior to the race so you can get it out of the way.

Most decent races will include a race T-shirt for you to keep after the race, and what is known as a "swag bag" with cool "merch" to take home. You can also use this bag to check some belongings with the race organizers prior to the start of the race that you may want in the finish area. The race sponsors will have your swag bag taken to the finish line for you to retrieve when you get there.

Another important item is a race timing chip incorporated in your number bib or one that you attach to your shoe. This allows accurate timing of your run when you cross electronic detection stations at the start and finish lines. Some races have devices at different intervals in the race to give you split times. You may even be able to sign up for a service that will send a text message to the phone of someone who is there to cheer you on and meet you at the finish. Technology is amazing, isn't it?

Regardless of the size of the event it is important to read all the information they give you to get yourself in the right place at the right time. Sometimes things change and what you thought was going to happen gets rescheduled, so pay attention.

Race Eve: What you do on the night before the race is as important as what you do on race day. It is particularly important to hydrate yourself well during the few days prior to the race but especially on Race Eve. If you are running a long race (60 minutes or more), eat a carbohydrate loaded meal (I like spaghetti) and eat early so you can get to sleep early. Do not experiment with a new recipe or try a new restaurant for your pre-race meal. Eat something that agrees with your stomach and do not overdo it. Eat a healthy meal that is filling but not bloating. I said carbohydrate loaded, meaning foods consisting of mostly carbohydrates, do not overload your stomach. Stay away from fried foods. Avoid drinking alcoholic or carbonated beverages if you can help it, they will detrimentally affect your effort on the run.

You will be nervous, and it may be hard to go to sleep, but get in bed early and stay there even if you find you are not sleepy. You will still be resting and eventually you will fall asleep. Set a good alarm. By this I mean use the alarm on your fully charged cell phone to wake you. If the electricity goes out in your home, or hotel room if you traveled for the race, then your cell phone will come through for you. These runs usually start early and you need to be up and at 'em even earlier.

You also want to get all your gear ready before you retire for the night. Shoes in place, number bib pinned to your shirt, runner's butt pack (or hydration pack, whatever you like) all set with everything you want with you during the race. There just will not be time in the morning – trust me. You may also want to put together your "after race" items to go into the swag bag. Think about what you might want at the finish; a dry shirt and/or socks to change into, lip balm, your favorite snack, a bottle of water for the smaller races (although I have never been in a race that didn't have some sort of hydration at the finish), and maybe a little cash (but not too much).

Race Morning: Reverse plan your wake-up time from the race start time to include time for eating something, dressing, and if necessary, driving to the start area. There may also be a designated shuttle pick-up area that you can use to get to the start line without having to drive into a traffic jam. You will have to know how long the transit to the start line is by shuttle so you can calculate your departure time from home or hotel. My suggestion is that you plan to arrive at the start line about 45 minutes to an hour prior to the start of the race. This will help if you encounter adverse traffic on the way to the race or if you are required to stand in line to get your number bib or perform any bodily functions before the running begins. I have found that I have a better run if I wake up at least two hours or more before the start time. You do not want to be half asleep when the gun goes off.

It is up to you if you want to eat anything before the race although I think it best to have a little something on my stomach when I run. I usually have a banana and water at least an hour before the start, so I wake and eat immediately, then get dressed. Light breakfasts are best before running and remember to hydrate, hydrate, and hydrate! Again, stay away from fried foods; maybe some toast or a bagel with your favorite spread will do. And you may find that brushing your teeth before running will give you "cotton mouth," so leave your toothbrush alone in the morning.

When it comes time to put your shoes on remember to slather your toes (and if necessary, your heels) with petroleum jelly before slipping on your socks to reduce friction during the run. Tie the laces loosely until just before you run so you do not restrict circulation too long beforehand. Once you are running the blood will flow, so a snug (but not too tight) shoe during the race will not make you uncomfortable. Snug the heel in well and tighten up for the long run.

In The Start Area: This is the most exciting time of the event for most people. You will probably have a bit of the pre-race jitters, which is normal. Even experienced runners will admit that just before the start, they are at least mildly nervous. Do not worry, when the horn blows, or the gun goes off, you will leave your nerves behind.

When you arrive at the start area you will have some work to do in order to be ready for the starter's gun. Take care of the administrative chores first by dropping off your swag bag and get in the port-o-potty line to drop off any internal stores before you warm up. Getting there early will help as there might be as many as 35,000 runners at the start, all wanting to do their business too. Once you have taken care of those things, you can start to prepare your body for the test to come. At this point I will pop some energy chews into my mouth to start the process of digesting what I will need in the next few hours.

Warming up and stretching is next. I use the same routine that I always use before every training run as discussed in Chapter 6. The only difference here is I take my time and really exaggerate every stretch to be sure I am totally loosened up. On race days I will also do about 5 – 10 minutes of light jogging to finish off the warm-up. This is also the time when I start to tune into my body to detect any anomaly both physically and mentally. This is really no time to be disconnected from yourself. It sounds silly, I know, but if you are processing an event in your past life while trying to prepare for the race, you will not run well. Let the world turn without you for a few hours. Focus on what is going on inside you in the present so you avoid inferior performance or, even worse, injury.

The Start Line: In the bigger races there will be "wave starts" where runners are divided into groups, or corrals, according to their anticipated finish times with a one-to-two-minute interval between the start of subsequent corrals. This kind of start helps to spread out the pack allowing runners to run faster from the beginning instead of slowly moving out like a herd of cows. And you do not have to worry about your start time being delayed. Your time will start when you, and your timing chip, cross the start line. Even so, you will want to wear a watch with a digital timer to monitor your pace as the race progresses. Remember to start it as you cross the start line.

In a wave start race, you will be all right anywhere in the corral, but as a beginner, you may want to move to the rear of the group and let everyone else take off in front of you. This way you can start with less distraction from people passing you. It is important to start slowly and gradually speed up to your pace. Be aware that you may get caught up in someone else's rhythm running at a pace that is too fast for you to start with. Run your race. The idea is to honor your training and finish the race, not to set any records. That comes later when you are working on your personal best run times. Avoid going out too fast and burning yourself out before you get into the race. Ease into the run and settle into your pace. You are on your way. Get comfortable and enjoy the event.

During The Race: Once you have attained your cruise velocity and are enjoying the run, stay conscious. There are lots of other bodies sharing the road with you. Some of them will not take care to be aware of you and will pose the threat of a collision, although most people will be watching out for others. There is nothing worse than taking a spill and twisting an ankle or biffing your knee on the pavement during a race. Act as if you are driving a car and check your blind spot beside you on either side if you decide to move to one side or the other on the course. I do not like to run on a sloping surface, so I am constantly looking for the most level section of road. Most city streets are constructed with a slope to the sides so water will run off and the level spots track either in the center or on the edge near the curb. At times I will move laterally to take advantage of the most level part of the raceway. Before I start my "lane change," I always look over my shoulder for someone overtaking me. I have had a few near misses, but it is usually when someone darts into my path as I am overtaking them. A word to the wise, leave as wide a berth as possible when passing slower runners. Most of the problems occur at the beginning and nearing the end of the race where people are in proximity, but most of the time things are spread out nicely for smooth sailing.

Water Stations: Every few miles, especially in longer races, there should be a hydration station featuring water and electrolyte drink. Race volunteers will be there to hand small cups containing either liquid. All you need to do is continue running and gently grab a cup. You can slow down slightly but whatever you do, do not stop completely to grab a cup. People behind you will run right up your back and bad things could happen at that point. If you miss the cup you are aiming for, go to the next person and get that one. There will be plenty of opportunities for you to get one or two cups of liquid in the station. Sometimes the drinks are just sitting out on the runner's side of the table and volunteers filling cups on the back side. So, you must snatch one from the group of cups sitting there. Most races have folks handing the cups to the runners; it is much easier. Throw the small amount of liquid down your throat, toss the cup to the side, and keep on trucking. On hot race days, you can throw a cup or two of water into your face or over your head to stay cool, that is legal. I carry my own electrolyte drink in my hydration pack, so I only hit the water stations. Do not overfill yourself - a little goes a long way. Also, start drinking at the first station - do not wait until you are thirsty before getting water, it will be too late then.

Fatigue Factor: In a run of 90 minutes or more you will hit "the wall" at some point. As your glycogen stores become depleted, you will become fatigued, and you will slow down. We talked about the energy chews being a help in replenishing some electrolytes and carbohydrates during the run. Some races will have a "GU" station where race volunteers pass out an energy gel supplement for all runners wanting them. Just like at the water stations, the name of the game is grab and go!

Remember to breathe properly. Even if you have enough energy to burn, you will become fatigued and slow down if you are not breathing properly. It is important to know at what pace you can continue to run and recover your breath. When you get to the point where you feel tired, slow down and catch your breath. It is fine to walk a short distance if you must but catch your breath and prepare for the push to the finish.

As you near the finish line, you should be pumped up and able to finish strong. Here is where the training pays off. If you remember all the things you learned about running during your workouts, you should be feeling good about getting to the finish. If you are completely drained at the end of the run, you will know better next time what you need to finish in good fashion. Train well, stay focused during the race and you will do fine. It is all about finishing.

The Finish Area: When you cross the finish line you will enter a "finishers only" area where you can get water, some nutrition (usually bananas or energy bars) and first aid if you need it. This is also the area where you will receive your finisher's trophy, usually a medal or a certificate, and get your picture taken. If you ran with friends, it is time for congratulations and relief as you leave the finisher's area. Do not forget to meet up with spectators who have come to see you finish. There should be a family, or a reunion area separated alphabetically for ease of finding folks in a crowd. This may be where the swag bag recovery area is as well.

It is a great feeling to have your first race under your belt. You can give yourself a big "high five" and enjoy the accomplishment. Now that you know what it is all about you can start preparing for the next event. But first, you will want to take a day or two off and let your body recover. In the post-race period, it is important to remember to hydrate, stretch, and hydrate some more. A liberal application of ice to the sore spots may be welcomed too. You worked hard getting there; it is all right if you pamper yourself for a while. Just do not slip back into the couch potato posture again.

Chapter 8: Your Motivation; Why Do This?

Outside of the obligations we agree to, there is only one reason to choose anything in life: for the fun of it. We all have things we have to do to survive or to help someone else survive and sometimes we are in a situation that we do not really like or want to continue necessarily. You may have heard the saying, *"You do what you have to do until you can do what you want to do."* That is not a bad philosophy, but who determines the time when you can do what you want? You do, of course.

The bigger question is, "How do I know what I want?" For me, that question is easy to answer; I do what makes me happy. Now I know some of you out there are thinking, *"What if doing something bad makes me happy? – are you saying I can do what I want to do without caring for the consequences? – can I kill my neighbor's dog that barks all night because I will sleep better and that will make me happy?* No, I am not saying that! Without going into a lesson on morals, I believe that we can all do what we want to do if it will not hurt or otherwise deprive someone else of their opportunity to be happy. And truly, I do not think I would take on long distance running, or any exercise regimen, because it was "good" for me, or because I would "look better." I do it because it makes me happy, it makes me feel better. When it ceases to be fun, I am sure I will stop doing it. Seeking joy in life is what we all need to do. In this chapter I am going to share some of the stories that illustrate why I do this.

It was in early November 2010 when I got the call from my eldest daughter, Cailin, who was living in Scottsdale,

Arizona, asking if I would join her in Phoenix for a half marathon in January 2011.

"Are you crazy, you're not a runner," was my initial thought. That was my "reasonable self" talking. If you remember my introduction to this book, I told you that I was in the worst shape of my life. My initial thought came from the viewpoint that I had never run more than three miles with any regularity before in my life. In the Marines we were required to do a physical fitness test twice a year consisting of doing pull-ups, sit-ups, and a three-mile run. To receive a maximum score on the test a Marine had to do twenty pull-ups, eighty sit-ups in two minutes, and the three-mile run in 18 minutes or less. I could do the pull-ups and the sit-ups, but, except for a few times when I was younger and lighter, the 18-minute pace was tough for me. I usually ran a 20:30 on average, which was still a high First-Class performance.

Running three miles in that time for a guy my size (I was 235 to 240 pounds on average then) was rather good, but I did not consider myself a "runner." I was a football player in college, and that type of running, as in most sports, except for running track events, involves short sprints of not more than forty yards and back to the huddle providing a nice rest. For a lineman, the requirement for running forty yards on a play was rare during games as the average run went from three to five yards and pass plays were usually beyond our capacity to catch up to in order to block someone anyway.

During the conversation with my daughter, I realized that I was limiting myself because of some belief I had formed years before about my running ability. Like a shot in the head, I received guidance that I was deciding not to participate in life because I thought I could not do it. Now mind you, there are some circumstances where doing this sort of thing would not be advised. I could have had some medical condition, or an "old football injury" that could have kept me from participating. But alas, I had no real "reason" to say no to my darling daughter. I would have to make one up to get out of this, and I just did not want to lie to my kid. I could have simply said "I don't want to do that," to try and escape, but she would have asked "Why not?" I did not have an answer to that, so I heard myself saying, "Sure Kid, I'll give it a go." Anything short of that would have felt like saying, "I don't want to participate in your life," and I could not imagine saying those words to her.

I had just under two months to prepare; about six- and one-half weeks to be exact. I decided to do some research and find a workout routine aimed at getting ready to run half marathons. There are plenty of "experts" out there, all with great advice for people of all abilities and conditions. In Chapter 10 I will share with you the program to which I gravitated. For now, just know that I selected an attainable workout for a person in my condition and started to run.

Oddly enough, by the time I got to Phoenix in January, even though I was making some progress with the new diet, I had not lost a significant amount of weight, eight to ten pounds or so (I had not fully modified my diet yet as described earlier). So, at just a shade under three hundred pounds and in marginal physical condition built up over a very short six weeks of not very intense exercise, I was standing at the starting line of my first half marathon.

I had set my goals for this event as; 1) running the entire distance non-stop and 2) finishing in three hours or less. As I revealed earlier in this book, I attained both of those goals. I ran a time of 2:45:48 and did not stop running until the finish line. I was dead on my feet and had surely hurt myself by pushing that far without being really prepared. But I did it and that is all that mattered.

One might ask why I would continue this torture after having such a tough first event. I was thinking the same thing when I was crossing the finish line. I figured this was my first, and last, half marathon, or run of any distance. About a half mile from the finish, I was passed by a guy wearing a T-shirt that said, "Never mind finishing, at my age, just starting is enough." He looked a bit older than I was at the time and I got a small kick out of that shirt which kept me moving just enough to make the finish line. In the runner's area at the finish, I caught up with him as he was grabbing a water bottle from the ice barrels provided. I turned to him and told him what an inspiration his T-shirt was for me. Then I said, "If you do not mind me asking. How old are you?" I thought he would say sixty-five or there about.

"Young fella," he said, "I'll be 79 until next Thursday."

I almost hit the ground in astonishment. Here was a man running 13.1 miles, and faster than I did, who was nearly 80 years old. He was 25 years my senior. At that moment, I knew that I would pursue long-distance running for the rest of my life, God willing. But I also knew I would have to prepare better for future runs than I had for that one. What a lesson for me in that tiny moment of grace with a fellow runner. I hope I meet up with him again.

After running several half marathons, I met some interesting people along the way, both in the events and during training runs. One of the more inspiring characters I have met along the way is "Charlie" (not his real name), a wounded warrior. Charlie was a veteran of the Afghanistan campaign who encountered an Improvised Explosive Device (IED) while on patrol in the Helmand Province with the U. S. Marines. He shared his unit with me, but I am going to keep that to myself for his privacy and for the others of his unit who befell a similar fate.

Suffice to say, Charlie and I met during one of the events I had entered. I could tell he was a Marine by looking at him, which is usually true for Marines even after they have left the service; they have that "look." Besides that, he had a beautiful Eagle, Globe, and Anchor emblem tattooed on his upper arm. I first saw him from his right side and as I approached to say, "Semper Fi Marine, good luck on the run," he turned to regard me. As he turned, he revealed a missing left arm from the elbow down and a prosthetic limb from the left knee down. It was one of those metal prosthetics that look like a car leaf spring made for running. Of course, I tried not to notice and greeted him as I would any of my Brother Marines, but I just could not help but ask where he had served and how it was for him to be there at an event like that.

"I can motivate pretty well with this thing," he said, pointing to the prosthetic limb attached to his lower leg. The word "motivate," when used in this manner, is Marine speak for "move" or "run." And then he said something that really got me as he read my expression.

"No regrets at all, really. Actually, I have less body to supply with blood now, so it sort of helps my run time."

I am guessing that it must surely have been a tongue-in-cheek statement which demonstrated a positive attitude about the starkness of the reality he now faced. Where do we get such people? God bless you Charlie and keep on running. You are truly an inspiration in anyone's book.

My running experience has allowed me to visit some places that I may never have had occasion to visit if not for a running event. I have seen some beautiful country, some magnificent sunsets, and sunrises while training. Being outdoors is incredibly special to me. I cherish the time I spend breezing through a park somewhere or an historic site where there is a running path to follow. One of my favorite places is along the George Washington Memorial Parkway, south of Alexandria, Virginia.

Starting from Mount Vernon, George Washington's home on the Potomac River, I would head north along the scenic pathway toward Alexandria, some eight miles away. With mile markers set out along the way, I can easily pick a turn-around point and head back to my car to accomplish my training objective. Sometimes I would ask a friend to meet me in Old Town Alexandria for lunch, after which they would assist me with a ride back to my car parked at Mount Vernon.

The run along the Potomac is just spectacular, full of scenes that take me back through the rich history of the region. I often think of the British warships that sailed past this area on the way to burn Washington in the War of 1812. About five miles or so north of Mount Vernon is River Farm, formerly of George Washington's estate and now the home of the National Horticultural Society. The mansion there is beautifully adorned with some of the most colorful flower beds ever planted.

One day as I was running along a section of the pathway that was adjacent to a neighborhood with some genuinely nice homes, I encountered two young girls who had set up a lemonade stand. I thought at first that they should not be there for their own safety until I saw that their mothers were watching them from the backyard not fifty feet away. Apparently, they were doing a Girl Scout project. As I ran by, they pleaded with me to stop and buy some lemonade. I told them I would be back and kept running. On my return, about 20 minutes later, I stopped as they made their cry for a customer once again.

"Have you sold any lemonade yet?" I asked.

"No, we just started, and you are the only one who has come by," they told me.

I felt for them, but I did not have any money. I told them that I would bring some money with me on my run the next time I ran by there. I was about to start running again when one of the moms walked down to the stand and said, "Give him a drink girls, he looks thirsty. He can pay you next time."

"OK, here you go," said one of the girls as she handed me a cup of lemonade.

I downed the cup, thanked the girls and their mom for their kindness, and asked what I owed them. Fifty cents was the agreed price, and I promised to stop by next time and pay my tab. "I hope you get more customers," I said. With that, off I went, telling everyone I passed coming the other way to buy some lemonade when they got to the stand.

The next week came, and I ran up the path anticipating a cup of lemonade with some money in my runner's pouch. As I rounded the corner and the stand came into sight, there were several people buying drinks. *"Great,"* I thought, *these kids are going to be happy."*

When I stopped to pay my debt and buy another cup, the mom who had suggested I get a free cup last time stepped up and told me, "This one is on the house too, you did some advertising last week for us and we owe you." I guess all the "shout outs" I made while running by people the previous Saturday churned up some business for them. A few of them had mentioned that "some runner" told them about the stand, and they decided to go far enough to find some refreshment.

"Really," I said, "well, I am glad to help the Girl Scouts. My youngest daughter earned her Gold Award doing stuff like this." I made a "donation" to the cause with the few bucks I stashed in my pouch, thanked the girls again, and went on my way. When I passed by there on subsequent runs, if they were there selling lemonade, they would get up with a cup and hand it to me as I passed by without stopping and I would drop a dollar on the table for their service to me.

If you go out there with the feeling that it is drudgery, that is what you will get. If you go out looking for adventure, you will get that too. It is up to you. I learned to enjoy all the fun I could get out of running. In the next chapter we will talk about the spiritual guidance afforded by this type of activity and explore the inner game of running.

Chapter 9: The Inner Game

In the last chapter I talked about the "little graces" that pop up while we are working on this activity. Anytime you spend working on yourself, you will encounter the small but powerful lessons of what the Universe has in store for you. At each turn in our road through life, we have a choice. We can choose a negative posture or a positive one. That is easily said and has little meaning for most of us. But the fact is if you say you can, or that you cannot, you will be right in both instances.

How does this apply to what we are talking about here? Aside from the simplistic idea that it is better to be happy than sad, or that it is better for you to maintain a positive attitude, I would like to open a discussion of the process we must go through to change anything in our lives. As I mentioned earlier in this book, we are mostly creatures of habit; both good and bad. As for that, there are no good and bad habits, there are just habits. Some habits lead us on a path of health, wealth, happiness, etc., and other habits lead us in a different direction.

Life itself is neither "good" nor "bad;" it is just life. For the same reason there is no "normal" life; there's just life. Now, this is not a "stuff happens" lecture where I tell you that you must be satisfied with everything you do or encounter in your life, or that you must tough it out, turn the other cheek, and endure things. This is about doing something about the situation. To begin the discussion, I must give some background into my thinking.

As you already know, I have spent a good deal of my life doing big and bold things in the world. I played Division

1 college football; I flew helicopters for the U. S. Marines; I jumped out of airplanes; I have hiked the high sierra mountains in California alone for days on end. In each case there was an element of physical risk, even danger, which I learned to manage and survive. But my spiritual self was not so big and bold. I played quite small spiritually in many situations. Maybe it was because I had no fears, or very few, in the physical world that I neglected my development spiritually. I am not saying that I had no spiritual foundation or that I was morally depraved, I am saying that I was unconscious to my spiritual being. In essence, I could not access nor benefit from the self that was hidden behind my eyes.

I am quick to say that I do not yet have it mastered, but I am working each day to become more aligned with the source of my being. Since I am physically oriented, I choose physical activities in which to explore my spirituality. It is not necessary to sit in a quiet place to be able to meditate and access a moment of grace from the Universe. Some of us access this part of our being through art, or music, or any number of other activities. The point is no matter what crayon we pick from the box; we can express our souls by coloring our world as we see it. There is nothing wrong with picking different crayons at different times to get your story out there. Don't have a story you say, of course you do, it is just lying dormant inside you, waiting to take its place among the world's greatest stories.

By "stories" I mean the expression of your soul, the sharing of who you are in the Universe of souls. Some souls are able to express themselves in a grandiose way. Most of us live our lives quietly expressing who we are and living vicariously through those who are able to express themselves boldly. That is why we have actors, politicians, and sports heroes. It is wonderful to have something to which you can look for enjoyment or fulfillment in some fashion, but that is not enough. We all need to shine in the world. We all need to be in touch with the source of our being. To the degree that you are conscious of the source of your being, is the degree to which you are able to access the power of your soul.

But how do we communicate with our souls, with the source of our being, or the Universe, or God, if you will? Those of us who pray may wonder about the answer more than the prayer itself. We wonder if our prayers are answered, or that we sometimes get a "no" for an answer to our prayers. If you are a person who does not think in terms of prayers, then you may wonder what effect you may have on the destiny that awaits you in this world or the next. If we are unpracticed at perceiving the answers to prayers, then how could we know if a prayer is answered?

The Universe, or God, or Source Energy, answers every prayer immediately. And the answer is always, "Yes!" How can that be true if "bad" things happen to people? Certainly, they do not pray for something terrible in their lives. I do not know of anyone who prays for cancer, and yet some people who pray get cancer. If the answer is always "Yes," why would the Universe, or God, or Source Energy, give a negative outcome when we ask for a positive one.

It is because the inner game, the subconscious mind, is at work all the time. Though we may make a conscious prayer asking for grace, our subconscious is outbidding those prayers in asking for things. Some things are a result of an unconscious "truth" or "belief" we have incorporated in our foundation. As it compares to prayer, our subconscious mind is working overtime sending out messages to the Universe, or God, or Source Energy, about everything we think, feel, or imagine. Unless we are in conscious prayer 24 hours a day, we will never outdo the communication from our subconscious mind to the Universe.

Remember the subconscious mind when I mentioned habits? In the case of an undesirable habit, it is merely a matter of what is easy and feels good to you that wins-out over "doing the right thing." So why not turn that subconscious mind into an ally to get what we want? Every thought we have has power in the Universe. The words we say are expressions of thoughts and, therefore, are powerful too!

The fears we have, whether about real or perceived threats to our existence, are even more powerful. Since our thoughts influence feelings, we must use caution in our daily thinking process. The saying, *"Be careful what you wish for, you just may get it,"* comes to mind. And truly, we get everything we wish for through our thoughts and feelings.

So that is how we communicate with the Universe and the Universe responds by giving us what we ask for, or more correctly, what it perceives we are asking for. If we are not consciously clear and aligned with what we genuinely want, the Universe will read the signals of our inner vibrations to decide what to give us. If we are praying for a miracle to happen in some life situation on the conscious level and we are fearful and focus subconsciously about not having what it is we are praying for, the Universe reads our focus, bringing us more of what we fear. Instead of focusing on not having, we can help ourselves by focusing on what we have and vibrating on a different level. Perhaps we should start with being grateful for what blessings we do have.

The Law of Attraction is based on vibrational energy. It is a physical reality that when something vibrates of a certain frequency, it attracts other things that vibrate the same way. If you had a room filled with tuning forks of all different frequencies, and you strike one tuning fork, making it vibrate, all the other tuning forks in the room of that same frequency will begin to vibrate and the others will not. In the same way our souls vibrate and attract similar souls or situations vibrating on the same frequency.

For example, imagine if our vibrational energy was like Scotch whisky. There are distinct brands and qualities of whisky from rotgut to the most well-aged and the smoothest kind. If you vibrate on the level of rot-gut whisky, you will attract rot-gut whisky people and situations. If you vibrate like a middle of the road whisky, you will attract the same. And if you vibrate like the finest single malt with the smoothest taste, you will attract top-level people and events into your life. As we change our vibrations, we will move to different levels of existence, hopefully for the better, but that is up to the individual. Our thoughts and feelings about the situations we face show how we are vibrating at any particular time. The Universe is a tuning fork of sorts that matches our vibrations, high or low.

As we have heard, "Success begets success." Successful people usually move from one success to another. When they encounter a failure, they do not look at it as failure;

they see it as a learning opportunity and move on. Less successful people are not able to see the positive side of the learning curve and are not able to move on so easily. They will focus not on their successes, but on the less successful parts of their lives. They energize their vibrations in feelings about failure, which is an emotional event in their lives. The Universe sees those vibrations as a "prayer" for more of the same and will send it straight away.

How does all this tie into a new health regimen? Well, you may agree with the idea that if you are in good health, you will feel well, and if you are feeling well, you will naturally vibrate on a higher level than if you are unhealthy. That alone will set you on a path to more enjoyment of your life creating a happier you. A happier you will create higher vibrations for the Universe to match. I am not saying that you will not encounter some situation that will cause concern, you will, but it is how you perceive the situation that creates the vibration in you, not the situation itself. By practicing good health habits, you will have less to vibrate negatively about, allowing you to focus on positive outcomes rather than the less successful situations you encounter.

That is how we communicate with the Universe, but how does the Universe communicate with us; again, by feelings. When we make decisions that are not right for us, we will get immediate feedback. We may not correctly perceive the feedback, or we may choose to ignore the feedback given us, but it is there, nonetheless. Have you ever had the feeling that someone in your life was not good for you? Regardless of whether they were an intimate relationship or just a casual acquaintance, you could feel the drain in your energy when they were around. You might call that feeling a mismatch in the vibrational energy between you and that person, but it is definitely a message to you that things are not right. The conscious person will take action and leave or address the situation to affect a remedy for the energy loss. The unconscious person will blame someone else or put the blame on something else for the situation they are experiencing, allowing the situation to persist.

What I am talking about is consciousness and your ability to tap into the inner self, a most powerful ally. You will not be in control of your inner self, your soul, if you do not practice, just as you will not run very well unless you train. As we know, our bodies are incredible machines, capable of doing some amazing things. Most of the time it is our minds that hold us back physically. Remember when I was discussing how our bodies react to a drastic change in our diet? I said our bodies would try every trick in the book to get us back to our old eating habits. In truth, it is the subconscious mind we are battling at that point. If we had an expert medical person or dietician telling us to expect the aches, pains, and cravings that we are having after starting our new lifestyle and that everything was all right with us, our subconscious mind would not make up terrible stuff about what our bodies were going through. It is all perception. Training creates a new perception in us. Once we run a half marathon, or even a 5K event, it is not so scary anymore. Once we tune into the effects of our subconscious mind, we can begin to train ourselves to be in control by making conscious decisions.

Part of my spiritual training involves addressing things while I am on a run. Without the motivation of being at an exciting event, I must make myself do the run training.

Sometimes, even now as I run, if I am not really in the mood, my subconscious mind will work on me to get me to stop running. *"You don't have time today; you'll be late for that appointment if you go that far; blah, blah, blah!"* I am good at compartmentalization, which means that I can ignore that stuff fairly easily. But when the subconscious cannot win that way, it starts to work on the physical twinges. Something will not feel right, and I will begin to think about that while running. I must be careful because I do not want to run with something that is a real physical ailment, such as a small strain. A small strain in your leg, for example, can turn into a big pull in a hurry. As mentioned previously, it is much better to not run one day, or to stop early on a training run, than to have to lay-off due to a pulled muscle.

So, I am constantly practicing being conscious of my body and what it is up to and battling the sub-conscious mind telling me things are going wrong. In every run I will get a twinge of some sort, perhaps an ache in my leg or a stitch in my side. The first thing I do is ask the feeling to go away. I will actually touch the spot that is bothering me and pretend that I am drawing out the pain into my fingers. Then I make a tossing motion with that hand as if I am throwing the pain away. I will then ask myself to relax and allow the feeling to leave me. Most of the time, that is all it takes, and I do not have to stop running to get that result. When the pain persists beyond a few minutes, I take a break and investigate it more thoroughly. Maybe I did not stretch out well enough or I am just carrying a bit more tension in my body. A few seconds of stretching and sometimes massaging of the area in question puts me back on the run. If the feeling persists past that point, I will stop the run, walk back to the car or my house, and call it a day.

The idea here is to make a conscious decision about what I am doing at all times. Being able to communicate with my subconscious mind and bridge the gap between mind and body is helpful to me in keeping my vibrations at a high level. It has always been a quest of human beings to draw a balance between the mind and the body. The idea of wellness is meant to address the mental, emotional, and physical aspects of our being. Leaving any of these pieces out would give us less than optimal health. These entities work together as they do their separate duties. Without the thought that I needed to make a change in myself, I could never have started or maintained a workout regimen of this nature or of any type.

So, my mind's desire for something new led me to the running program I have adopted. Since starting this regimen, my consciousness has become more acute, not only within myself, but of the world around me as well. I have always fancied myself as a person who could hold to the lofty ideals in my mind. I also have been a person who could create things in my world through the use of art, woodworking, sports, writing, etc. Until I started my new lifestyle, beyond losing weight or the improvement in my physical condition, I was less able to plug into the creative things as I was less conscious of the entirety of my being.

Things did not come to me as easily as they do now. It is as if I have gotten a tune-up along the way making my creative engine run stronger and more smoothly. In a word, I "flow" a bit more than I used to. My younger daughter, Colleen, has been a wonderful teacher for me to understand "flowing" in the Universe. Now I can recognize patterns in my life, both beneficial and detrimental, which were difficult for me to see before. It is not just from becoming more fit, for I have been in much better shape in my past, it is drawing into balance my physical and spiritual being.

The divine paradox of the accumulated experiences of my life is a validation of something greater than myself in the Universe. Some people call that God, some call it Karma, but however you address your experience of the power of consciousness, the common thread is that it binds humankind together and that we are all in on it. We are all a part of a universal consciousness, and what is more, it is a part of us. I use the word paradox in describing my existence because my personal composition is drawn from different worlds. As big as I was on the outside, my inner self was small. By this I mean that I was out of balance spiritually with my outside manifestation in the Universe. I exercised my physical being much more than my spiritual being. And that was my choice. There was nothing stopping me from developing my inner skills, I just left them alone.

There is paradox as well in my life experiences from the viewpoint of what I chose to do. It is not typically known that physical beings like football players and Marines can be spiritual in their nature. They do not usually show that side of themselves, but it is there. I was never aware of it during my days on the gridiron or in the Corps, but I was at my best when I thought creatively and on a much more energetic level. I did not acknowledge that part of myself as it was not typical for anyone in either of those communities to have an individualized approach. They were, strictly speaking, team-oriented families. In essence, I was unable to develop my spiritual side as I was completely unconscious of the power it held for me. When my spiritual nature would appear, I simply disregarded it as contrary to the purpose of the group.

You could say that at times my spiritual side was at work, but I did not recognize it.

Before exercising my spiritual being I was unable to see the small graces that came as little gifts to me, teaching small lessons that could have had a much greater effect on my life. Being more conscious that these graces are there at every turn allows me to look for them and more easily see them. As I practice "seeing" them, I get better at recognizing more of them. The remarkable thing is I did not miss anything because these lessons will keep coming back again, and again, until I learn them. Then they can go away. Now I see graces that take me back to my past at a time when I missed the lesson. I have a storehouse of memories that have given me the knowledge of having traveled that road, or something similar, more than once.

When I get to running and the rhythm of my footfall matches with my breathing, it is as soothing as when I am quietly meditating in my favorite room at home. Both these methods of reaching the inner game are equally powerful for me. There again is another paradoxical situation where one method supports the other in getting to the self I seek. Even the idea of running and relaxing at the same time during the run is yet another paradox. But I can tell you that my best runs are the ones where I am completely relaxed, all the tension is gone from my body, and I am flying along at a good clip as if I were not in my body but floating above the trail or bike path. It is a wonderful feeling and one that I seek every time out. The more I run, the more I get into that trance-like state of mind, fully aware, but totally relaxed and in the zone. Oh, the places you can go to while you are in the zone.

Chapter 10: Last Words and Helpful Tools

It is time to wrap things up and say, "Adios mi amigo." But before I go, I want to share a few things that will assist you in your journey down this road. Hopefully, I have given you enough information to enable you to know whether this is something you want to do yourself. Aside from me pointing to running as an activity to make the leap into a healthy condition, I think the nutrition information should at least set you in the right direction should you want to make a change there. And I highly suggest everyone get their diet under control.

A few last words about what I told you and to refocus on the point of this book are in order here. First, let me say once again, this is my story with some factual data sprinkled in. I am not an expert in this field, but I do have experience that you may learn from, and I hope you did just that. Also, you must consider that even the "experts" differ in opinion about what is happening in the human body when it comes to diet and exercise. Sure, there are generally known things that have been tested and found to be reliable in explaining the processes involved in the study of health issues. Just remember it is up to you to investigate for yourself what works best for you. Take my word for it; you cannot take anyone's word for anything when it comes to your health. You have got to be at least a partner in the care and feeding of your body and soul.

As a further warning about information you may hold to be the "truth," you need to be careful with what you know or think you know about any subject. What may be ingrained in your head about how the world is could be information that does not serve you very well. Sometimes there is some truth to the "old wives' tales," and sometimes they hold no validity in your world at all. It does not have to be an old wives' tale to be misinformation in your head either. Sometimes we will formulate opinions and responses to situations based on old or bad information that we "learned" over the years. Even if it was true then, it does not make it true now. So, my guidance is to continually refine your base of knowledge and be sure to check the old way of thinking at the door.

In checking yourself for faulty processes working within you, the best way I know to start is to examine every word that comes out of your mouth. Remember, ingrained habits die hard. The way we refer to things in our lives is as important as what we have to say. One of the best changes I made to my speech patterns at the suggestion of a dear friend of mine was to stop using the phrase, *"I love it to death."* I know that phrase is used to accentuate the degree to which you love something, and it means you love something a lot. But why love it to death? Why not love it to life? It is a small thing, but it makes a big difference.

Suffice to say that we have learned cute little quips to describe things about us or our loved ones. I used to say things like, *"Not a bad run, for an old guy."* If you think about it, that statement indicates that I am not happy with my run because I am qualifying it in such a way as to tell the Universe I am old, or at least I am running slower than when I was young. We know that is true, but to reinforce it only drags you down. Now I say things like, *"I had a fantastic run,"* or *"I ran faster than ever."* It is the little things that count.

Next, I would like to share my method of tracking my progress during training and my overall progress for the runs I choose. I have gathered some other resources for your use. These are not meant to be the definitive answers for all questions on running, but they will launch you in the right direction. When I started to track my progress, I constructed an Excel spreadsheet with a 12-week training period based on the plan I got from Hal Higdon's website. If you are an Excel person, you can do the same. There is also a race tracking block at the conclusion of the training for you to log your performance during the events in which you run.

There are many, many more resources out there. Just let yourself wander through all the amazing websites, magazines, and books out there. Try this site first:

http://www.halhigdon.com.

Hal's website provides all you will need to get started running and preparing for any level of running event from 5Ks to marathons. I recommend reading as much as you can by Mr. Higdon, especially if you are a beginning runner. He offers a downloadable app so you can run with him on your phone. Here you will find everything from sports nutrition, training tips, gear reviews, and more featured on this site.

The next site will give you all the information about the Rock N Roll running group and their events world-wide. Check it out.

http://www.runrocknroll.com

This is where you can look for more race event info:

http://www.active.com

Do some research on the Internet to find more than you will need in the way of advice, tips, and assorted information.

Lastly, I want to leave you with a checklist for preparation on race day. After all the training you will do to get ready, the last thing you want is to forget something that will make your race day successful and fun.

Event Checklist

1. Pick an event that you can finish.

2. Register for your selected event as soon as you are able.

3. If you register online, download all the race day information and read it carefully.

4. Pick up your race packet early (preferably the day before).

5. Be sure to review your packet materials for any changes to the race-day information.

6. Eat a carbohydrate loaded meal the night before the race (especially for half marathon and up) and eat early.

7. Set up your race-day clothing the night before: number bib pinned on your shirt, all your gear laid out, Vaseline at the ready, racer's timing chip in place.

8. Think about your hydration plan. Fill water bottles, hydration pack, etc.

9. Put your electrolyte and/or energy gel in your runner's butt pack.

10. Set an alarm independent of the electric grid (watch or cell phone works nicely)

11. Get to sleep early.

12. Wake up at least two hours prior to the start time. Earlier if you have to account for travel time.

13. If you need to eat something light, make time for that as well. Reverse plan from start time.

14. Be sure to put Vaseline on all friction areas of your body as you dress; toes (or more of the feet if necessary), crotch, armpits, and nipples (saves them from soreness later).

15. Be in the start area at least 1 hour prior to the start time.

16. Take care of the Swag Bag and get into the port-o-potty line.

17. Stretch out and warm up thoroughly before you get to the start line.

18. Retie your shoes for a snug fit and double knot them so they will not loosen during the run.

19. Have an enjoyable run and finish!!

Once your first event is finished, you will be an "old hand." You will know what works for you and what does not. Keep refining your preparation for the next event to get things just as you like them. Most of all, you should have fun doing this. If you track your progress, you will enjoy it more each race event you enter.

Remember, this writing should serve only as a beginning for you as you embark on a new adventure. To move on you must pick up the ball and run with it in terms of finding out what is new in this community. Keep abreast of new techniques, gear, etc. that will help you perform better in years to come. I wish you a long, happy life and enjoyable running! Thank you for reading my book.

www.ingramcontent.com/pod-product-compliance
Lightning Source LLC
Chambersburg PA
CBHW070631130626
46555CB00006B/2519